Readers comments about
A YEAR OF MIRACLES

"A beautifully written book. Words that could only come from one in tune with their Spiritual Self. People need to know they possess the same strength within to create their own healing power. One of the best love stories I have ever read."
Dot S., Massage Therapist, PA

"My 13 year old daughter and I read a chapter together every day. It gives hope to both of us, and strengthens our belief in my ability to also heal from cancer."
Donna V., Cancer Patient, MI

"I have loved and known Susan for lifetimes... because to know Susan is indeed to love her. I met my friend in this lifetime during the most difficult challenge she faced... healing from the cancer that invaded her body. Susan made the choice to live... to choose life... through Divine Order, Love, and Light. In her book, *A Year of Miracles*, she shares with us her emotional highs and lows, her laughter and her tears, all of her experiences in her miracle year. Her book provides the reader with inspiration, hope, belief, and faith that indeed all things are possible through God. Make this book a definite choice to read."
Catherine "Chetana" Florida,
Founder of The Lighthouse Center, Whitmore Lake, MI

"Three cheers for Love, Optimism, and the fighting Spirit. Describing a blend of medical science and spiritual science, *A Year of Miracles* is a very personal and beautifully written story about the journey of a spiritual warrior, battling with the self on the path to healing and wholeness from a form of cancer considered by many to be terminal. In the midst of a possible death sentence, Susan Wolf Sternberg created the life she wanted to live. Trusting in God as the source of all good, awakening her own Inner Physician, using patience and perseverance, she journeyed beyond old limitations, becoming an active participant in her healing, rather than being a passive victim of her disease. Cherishing each day as a gift not to be taken for granted, she makes crystal clear that there is no false hope, only false no hope. Reading this book is a must for anyone faced with the challenge of cancer seeking to strengthen the will to live."
James A. Thomas, M.D., Director, Behavioral Medicine and Oncology,
The Center for Contemporary Medicine, Ann Arbor, MI

"Your inspiring and beautifully written book has ignited a small flame beneath my will... to move forward... persist....and heal."
Chriss T., Nurse, CA

"Your book is extraordinary... should be required reading...truly a gift to all."
Lily Jarman-Rohde, Director of Field Instruction,
University of Michigan, School of Social Work, Ann Arbor, MI

"INSPIRATIONAL. Your words leapt out of the page and touched deep within my heart and soul. FAITH. That, for me is the driving message in your book."
Laura S., Meditator, and Lighthouse Center member, MI

"I just finished reading *A Year of Miracles*, and plan to send it with all my highlighted passages and notes on the borders, to my sister and mother who have recently been diagnosed with cancer. Thank you for taking the time to write your book. It truly moved me."
Carollee S., Nurse, CA

"When I first met Susan I didn't know that she had just completed her miraculous year of healing from cancer. What I did sense in her was a deep strength and courage, an abiding faith, and a warm and loving heart... all things she brought with her on her journey, and that were multiplied by it. Susan is a beautiful witness to all of us who have life and death struggles with the body, the heart, the mind, the soul. I recommend her book to my patients and friends, and to anyone who is struggling and needs a beacon of love and hope."
Nirmala Nancy Hanke, M.D., Psychiatrist, MI

"This book represents the true story of a very remarkable individual who has been able to survive an advanced stage of kidney cancer. Her tale is a poignant story of the emotional roller coaster which cancer patients undergo with their initial diagnosis and subsequent therapy. This very personal account will give readers insights into both the weaknesses and strengths of what medical practitioners can offer patients. I would strongly urge physicians, especially those who deal with cancer patients, to read this book in order to get a clearer understanding of the patient's perspective. I certainly learned a great deal."
Alfred E. Chang, M.D., Professor of Surgery.
Chief, Division of Surgery Oncology, University of Michigan Medical Center, Ann Arbor, MI

"Compelling. Moving. Courageous. A Celebration of Life."
Brenda F., Author, Public Relations Director, TX

"Can't put your book down. It has just grabbed me, and I have to keep reading."
Terri W., Hypnotherapist, Nurse, Cancer Survivor, CA

"Though I don't have cancer, nor do I work with many cancer patients, I am around hospice patients who have come to our facility to spend their last days. It is hard for me to watch their slow slide into the next world. I thought it would be good to read a positive story of cancer to balance myself, and to share with those around me. Thank you for your spirit and fortitude to have accomplished the impossible, and the grace to share it with the rest of us."
Anne P., Occupational Therapist, CO

"I will share your book with others in the hope that they can also benefit from your experience. I believe your positive mental outlook directly contributed to your having done so well."
Max Wicha, M.D., Director, University of Michigan Comprehensive Cancer Center, Ann Arbor, MI

"I read your marvelous book about your fight with cancer, as a fight against fear and pessimism.... with cancer providing the focus. I imagine that different people have different responses to your struggle. Mine is to focus on your ability to marshal so much support. In my spiritual practice I have gotten somewhat comfortable with asking help of God.... but it's odd that it takes a lot more consciousness to ask it of folks. So thank you for the gift of your example."
Jim A., Scientist, National Institutes of Health, MD

"A wonderful story...there is a flash of magic about it, and yet very practical, down to earth happenings and suggestions."
Gwendolyn Jansma, Ph.D., Author, Healer, CA

"I cannot express how happy I was to receive your book and learn of your conquering cancer. Your journey of faith, healing and medicine is very enlightening and inspiring. Thank you for sharing so much of yourself."
Grace Jordison Boxer, M.D., Hematology Oncology Associates of Southern Michigan

"Your story is one of tremendous courage and strength, coupled with unfailing love and support."
Beth S., Research Producer, CA

"Your book helped me realize how many miracles have already occurred in my life, and that makes it easier to have faith that the rest of my life will unravel according to God's plan. Though I have never had a terminal illness, I was able to relate the principles in your book to the adversity I have faced in overcoming a severely traumatic childhood. I am proud of the things I have already accomplished, and am confident that the best part of my life is still waiting for me. Just as you knew that one day you would be cancer free, I know that one day I will be healed from the wounds inflicted upon me as a child. Thank you for being a great teacher for me."
Carla H., Social Worker, MI

"I found true inspiration in Susan's book. I have shared it with others, and have referred friends and patients to her. *A Year of Miracles* has opened my eyes to the value of a positive mental attitude, an open mind, and hope in dealing with disease. I do not believe that I will ever view or treat patients with cancer in the same way as I did before reading Susan's book."
Mary Barton Durfee, M.D., Internist, MI

"Susan Wolf Sternberg has walked through the valley of the shadow of death, and emerged whole on the other side. Her book, *A Year of Miracles,* is compelling reading. The disbelief at the initial diagnosis, the physical pain from treatment, the 'raging and pleading with God,' the emotional rollercoaster of dealing with invasive cells ... they're all there. Susan is testimony to the power of mind over body, belief in God, and her own ability to take charge of her illness."
Don Faber, Staff Reporter, Ann Arbor News, MI

A Year of Miracles

A Healing Journey
from Cancer to Wholeness

Susan Wolf Sternberg

STAR MOUNTAIN PRESS

Ann Arbor

Book and Cover design by Simcha Wolf

Excerpts on pages 56 and 96 from *The Book of Runes* by Ralph
Blum, 1982 by Ralph Blum. Used by permission of St. Martin's
Press, New York.

Excerpt on page 121 from *Medicine Cards* by Jamie Sams and
David Carson, 1988 by Jamie Sams and David Carson. Used by
permission of Bear and Company, Santa Fe.

Library of Congress Catalog Card Number: 96-92246

ISBN 0-9653755-0-1

First Edition
Printed in USA
Printed on recycled paper

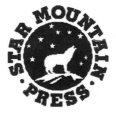

STAR MOUNTAIN PRESS
Post Office Box 1845
Ann Arbor, Michigan 48106
E-Mail StarMtnPrs@aol.com

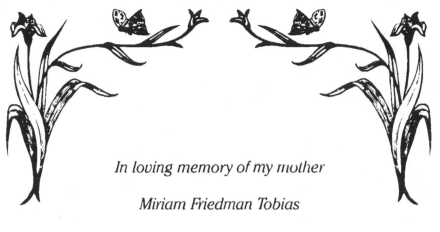

In loving memory of my mother

Miriam Friedman Tobias

June 16, 1913 - May 31, 1974

No matter what, she believed in me

for all the days of her life.

By believing in the best of me,

she helped me reach deep within

and discover the Source

from where all else flows.

DEDICATION

To my daughter Sharon Jill Hoeker, who walked with me every step of the way.

To my daughter Elyssa Kim Mount, who was always there when I needed her.

To my son Brent Ian Weiner, who made me laugh when I wanted to cry.

To Kal and Karen Tobias, who embraced me as only family can.

To Marilyn Winfield, who "worked her magic" in helping me heal.

To Susan Hanna Moss, whose unshakable faith nourished and sustained me.

To Dr. Alfred Chang, a gifted and dedicated physician and researcher.

To Dr. James Thomas, a compassionate healer who believed in me.

And especially ...

To Stanley Wolf Sternberg, my husband, my lover, my best friend, for his unconditional love, devotion, and unrelenting commitment to my healing.

ACKNOWLEDGEMENTS

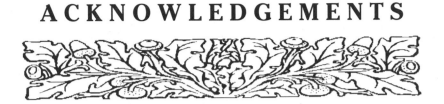

My heartfelt thanks to Sharon Jill Hoeker, Elyssa Kim Mount, Brent Ian Weiner, Jennifer Niedermeier, and Adrienne Anderson, who enthusiastically read the first draft of this book, and offered many thoughtful, constructive, and helpful suggestions, along with ongoing encouragement, love, and support.

I am grateful to June Gottleib, Susan Moss, and Marilyn Winfield, who eagerly listened as I read chapters of this book to them, applauding and encouraging me in this undertaking.

This book has only benefited from the proofreading skills of Lori Crall, and I am appreciative of the fine job she has done.

Many thanks to Brando, who was my constant companion, sharing my desk and keeping me company during the two years this book took form. You made a solitary task that much more enjoyable. As cats go, they don't come any better than you.

I am deeply indebted to my husband Stanley Wolf Sternberg for being ever present through the highs and lows while I wrote my book, and for knowing when to offer a kind word, a much needed back rub, or a shoulder to lean on. He willingly took upon himself the jobs of design and layout, graciously handling the necessary details, so that this book could find its way to those who need it the most. Stan, I love you forever and a day.

C O N T E N T S

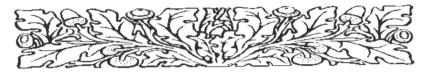

PROLOGUE:	*Firewalk*	3
CHAPTER 1:	*A New Year*	9
CHAPTER 2:	*First, the Bad News*	13
CHAPTER 3:	*Reaching Out*	19
CHAPTER 4:	*Diagnosis*	23
CHAPTER 5:	*Misdiagnosis*	29
CHAPTER 6:	*Emergency and Re-diagnosis*	33
CHAPTER 7:	*Angels of Darkness, Angels of Light*	39
CHAPTER 8:	*From Hope to Despair*	45
CHAPTER 9:	*Keep Your Spirits Up*	53
CHAPTER 10:	*I Shed My Light on Thee*	59
CHAPTER 11:	*Then Will I Perform Miracles*	71
CHAPTER 12:	*I Love You, I Love You, I Love You*	81
CHAPTER 13:	*There is No False Hope*	91
CHAPTER 14:	*Personal Best*	107
CHAPTER 15:	*Recurrence*	119
CHAPTER 16:	*I Choose Life*	133
CHAPTER 17:	*Healing From Within*	149
CHAPTER 18:	*A Healing Circle*	169
CHAPTER 19:	*Going for the Gold*	189
CHAPTER 20:	*And Now for the Good News*	201
EPILOGUE:	*Living the Miracle*	215
APPENDIX:	*Recommended Reading*	235

Believe nothing because a wise man said it,
Believe nothing because it is generally held.
Believe nothing because it is written.
Believe nothing because it is said to be divine.
Believe nothing because someone else believes it.
But believe only what you yourself judge to be true.

THE BUDDHA

A Year of Miracles

A YEAR OF MIRACLES

PROLOGUE

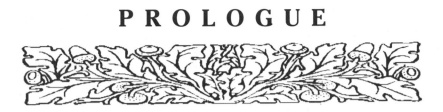

Firewalk

On March 31, 1992, almost a year to the day I was diagnosed with advanced terminal kidney cancer, which had metastasized to my hip, liver, second and seventh ribs, I learn all visible signs of tumor are gone from my body. I AM CANCER FREE. My yearlong journey toward healing and wholeness is fashioned out of hope and despair, courage and fear, faith and trust, laughter and tears, and an ongoing abundance of love, light, and miracles. I believe it is possible to accomplish the seemingly impossible. It is my hope that by sharing my story, you will come to see that even in the gravest of circumstances, you are free to choose your own attitude, and create your own path, as you journey toward healing and wholeness.

To begin with, I want to acknowledge I was blessed from the start. Long before I learned I had cancer, all the elements that needed to be in place were gathering. I was surrounded by loving, supportive family and friends, a strong belief in the goodness of God, work that fulfilled me, a budding relationship with a very special man, and an experience that had taught me it is possible to accomplish the seemingly impossible.

I was at a weekend retreat called The Way Of Our Grandmothers, with fifty other women in the Michigan wilderness. It was to be a weekend of renewal and growth. For me, it was transformative. As part of the weekend, I would have the opportunity to firewalk, which both attracted and repelled me. As a very young child I had been traumatized by fire, when in a violent act of rage, my father set my hair ablaze. Thirty years later I uncovered my first memory, and entered therapy to resolve the trauma. I knew instinctively, were I to firewalk, a complete healing would occur, that would irrevocably change my life. I desperately wanted to firewalk, but I was terrified.

On Saturday evening, I gathered with others in a solemn procession. Carrying logs to feed the blazing fire that would take four hours to burn to a bed of red hot coals, which would later be raked for the walk, I offered my gift of wood. I spent those hours intently listening as the firewalking instructor talked about knowing what is in harmony with your highest good, and honoring that knowing. Her basic premise was, if in doubt, don't. Until the last moment I was uncertain, but then I felt the knowing settle into my bones.

As I walked across the burning coals, I could hear the heels of my feet sizzling. As I stepped off the red hot coals, my feet were hosed down, and I could see the steam rising in long wispy streams. Though I examined them thoroughly, there wasn't a mark on either foot. There was nothing to show I had firewalked, except for some ash I gathered the next morning from the then cold fire to carry in a sacred pouch. But I don't need ash to remind me. The memory is imprinted within my body cells. They remember, and I remember that:

Six steps in six seconds
across burning coals
teaches me
it is possible
to accomplish
the seemingly impossible.

I don't know if it would have been different if I hadn't firewalked. I don't know if it would have been different if I didn't have love in my life. I don't know if it would have been different if I didn't have faith and trust in God, and a strong knowing that God wants me to live. If I didn't have a partnership with God, where God speaks and I listen, I just don't know. I don't know how I would have fared if I hadn't already made significant inroads toward resolving many of the traumas in my life, utilizing the lessons I was learning as an opportunity for new growth and healing.

The physical abuse, and subsequent abandonment by my father. The untimely death of my beloved mother. Divorce the following year at age thirty five. My near death experience barely three months later. Adjusting to being a single parent of three young children, and releasing guilt for "putting my children through the pain of divorce." The terror of being "entirely on my own," without another adult to depend upon. Returning to school, and obtaining a graduate degree in social work. Co-creating with four visionary women, a successful counseling center based on equal parts of faith, naiveté, and a burning desire to help other women in need. Buying our family home, and qualifying for a conventional mortgage. These experiences, and many others, strengthened, sustained, and helped shape me into the strong, independent, loving, spiritual woman who gradually emerged.

I can't give you a formula to use, as you journey toward healing from cancer or any other life threatening illness. I wish I could, but I can't. I can only tell you what I did, and hope that in the telling there are answers for you. Although your answers may be different from mine, it is my hope they help strengthen your belief in the possibility of accomplishing the seemingly impossible.

This is your life. Take as much charge of your illness as you can. Be an active participant, rather than a passive victim. Do research into both the traditional and alternative options available to you, and then choose the treatments that you believe in, and the doctors you feel trust in, because both are essential to your healing. I don't know how I would have fared without Dr. Chang and Dr. Thomas. I'm grateful I'll never have to know. But I do know that I asked. I questioned. I persisted. I wouldn't take no for an answer.

I refused to be treated by any doctor who would not offer me hope, and there were many. They were the doctors who would look at me with certain death in their eyes as they read my diagnosis; metastasized renal cell carcinoma, with secondary tumors infiltrating the hip, the liver, the ribs.

"Yours is an advanced terminal cancer," were the words I would hear. "The odds are heavily stacked against you, and you are not likely to survive. I would advise you to get your affairs in order now."

I dismissed every doctor who was convinced I was going to die. I heard what they said, and I knew what they believed, but I refused to lose hope, and I continued to look elsewhere.

I wanted a doctor who would work with me. One who would see me as a unique individual, rather than a statistic. A doctor who believed in me, as I believed in myself. A doctor who believed it was possible to accomplish the seemingly impossible. A doctor who was eager to try. I found that in Dr. Thomas and Dr. Chang. Two very different kinds of doctors, but both of them willing to go that extra mile. Wonderful healers. Caring compassionate men, whom God works through in healing and loving ways.

I encourage you to fight for your life, to give it your very best shot. Please don't allow yourself to lose hope and be stopped by words like "terminal." By words like "one year." "Metastasis." "Fourth stage." "No hope." "So very sorry." There are miracles. They happen all the time. Miracles are not dependent upon any particular belief system. They occur for the young and old, the rich and poor, those who believe in God, and those who don't. My healing is a miracle. If it happened for me, it can happen for you. I'm not more special, more important, more anything than you. I'm just another human being who values life. I want to lead a life where I can do some good, where I can enjoy, and be enjoyed by those I love, and who love me. Where I can be filled with God's love, share it with others, and live out God's plan.

I believe more than anything else, that I, like you, have my own unique qualities, but that I am just an ordinary person. Some people would disagree. Some people would say, you have healed from terminal cancer and that makes you special. I don't agree. I sometimes have an ego that is larger than I might like it to be, but most of the time it is well balanced. I don't think I'm exceptionally unique, and I don't consider myself unusually special. I do believe that the reason I am alive, the reason I am writing this book and sharing my story with you, is part of God's ongoing plan for me.

Since the word God occurs with some regularity throughout this book, I would like to share with you the reader what I mean when I speak of God. Despite growing up in an Orthodox Jewish household, and carrying the body knowledge of being a Jew, I do not follow the Jewish religion in a traditional sense, considering myself more spiritual than religious. I seldom attend synagogue, other than on the High Holy Days, and that has been so ingrained as to become part of my being. I cannot find the Divine, which is how I think of God, in any organized House of Worship. I couldn't as a child, and I still can't as an adult. I feel One with God when I am in nature. When I am in prayer. When I am giving thanks for the start of each new day. When I am in meditation. While I am hiking in the mountains, or resting under the sheltering branches of an ancient oak tree. I feel closest to God when walking along the ocean shore. Seeing an eagle in flight. Planting flowers in the moist Michigan soil. Praying to do God's Will, whatever that might be.

My spiritual journey has taken me into the world of Eastern thought and Zen Buddhism. Into Native American culture. To Jain meditation. To Spiritual Teachers, and Ascended Masters. To the study of the Goddess. To Tarot. The Kabbalah. The Viking Runes. The Medicine Cards. To many esoteric practices. From all of this I have come away with the belief in One God. To me the word God represents a whole field of creative energy which is Supreme and Divine. Masculine and Feminine. This God energy flows freely through me whenever I open myself to Its presence, and It is always centered in love. It communicates with me through visions, through dreams, through both written and spoken messages, through body knowing, through prayer, and in the silence of meditation. When I attentively listen to and honor this God energy, only good follows, and miracles frequently occur. I believe this same creative energy flows through all of us, Christian and Jew, Buddhist and Hindu, the pious, the agnostic and the atheist. If we were only to recognize this as truth, to know we are all connected, all part of the God energy, and therefore all children of God, imagine how different our lives and our world would be.

CHAPTER 1

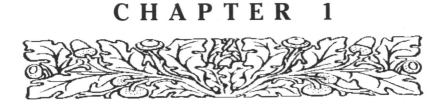

A New Year

Later I will call it the best of years and the worst of years, but on New Year's Eve as I joyously welcome 1991, I cannot, in my wildest dreams imagine what is about to unfold. Dreaming is something I do regularly, and not only at night. Since early childhood, I spend time daydreaming. As I grow to adulthood, I learn to take the steps necessary to change my dreams into reality. I don't know it at the time, but this creative ability is to become an essential tool in my fight for life. However, on January 1, 1991, my mind is engaged in far more pleasant pursuits.

I am in Toronto with Stan, a man I have been dating these past few months. The more time we spend together, the stronger my feelings for him grow, and I am looking forward to a deepening of our relationship. I feel alive, healthy, happy, and vibrant. My children whom I dearly love, are an ongoing source of comfort and pleasure. I am blessed with loving family and friends. My work as a psychotherapist in private practice at Tapestry Counseling Center fulfills me, and my partnership in Creating Results, a newly formed consulting business excites me. At fifty, my life is going wonderfully well. I have every reason to believe this will be a very good year.

On New Year's Day, as has been my custom for many years, I meditate and then draw a Rune Stone to represent an overview of 1991. The Runes, consisting of twenty-five differently marked stones, are an ancient Viking oracle used for divination. They can be used to evoke the knowledge of our Knowing Self, or what many refer to as our Higher Self. They can also be a means of communication between the

Self and the Divine. On that bright, clear, sunny winter day, I draw the Rune of Partnership. I interpret this as a sign that my relationship with Stan will deepen into a loving partnership. What I am blissfully ignorant of, is the deepening of the loving partnership between my Self and God that is about to unfold.

The first hint of trouble in paradise occurs towards the end of January. I am with women friends at Lily Tomlin's one woman show. As we walk down a long flight of steps, my left leg feels heavy and numb, and I experience intense pain in my groin. It lasts about a minute, but recurs several times over the next few hours. I don't pay much attention to it, and by the end of the evening it is gone. The following day, we celebrate my son Brent's twentieth birthday. Surrounded by the family I so dearly love, I am one happy woman. Having Stan by my side, only adds to my happiness.

At work a week later, my left leg and groin begin to ache. This time the discomfort continues, so I schedule an immediate appointment with the body worker I have been seeing. I feel somewhat better after the session, but the following day the pain intensifies, and I am unable to bear weight on my left leg. Feeling concern, and wondering if the body work may have reopened an old childhood injury involving my left leg and hip, I visit my primary care physician. After a thorough physical examination, my problem is diagnosed as deep muscle strain. My physician prescribes pain killers, crutches and physical therapy twice a week. We schedule a follow up appointment for early March.

With the start of physical therapy, I am exposed to a whole new world. My problem appears insignificant compared to the physical problems that other patients have. I find myself wondering if I would have the courage and strength to overcome such obstacles and challenges. I greatly admire the determination and perseverance these men, women, and children exhibit, and feel grateful to not be so challenged. As physical therapy continues, I experience some relief. The ultrasound and gentle stretching exercises appear to be helping. Physically, I am improving. I have discontinued all pain medication, walk using only one crutch, and can now bear some weight on my left leg. Encouraged, my physical therapist slowly adds an exercise bike and step climbing as part of my ongoing therapy. That weekend, the pain intensifies significantly. In desperation, I up my dosage of the medication, and once more begin using both crutches to move about.

"I overdid the exercise," I say to Stan when he expresses concern. "I did too much too soon. I should have taken it slower."

"It seems your leg should be stronger than it is," he replies.

Tears spring to my eyes, and my heart turns over in fear.

"Are you suggesting something more serious is happening?" I ask apprehensively.

"I don't know. Probably not. I just want you to be all right," Stan answers, and gently embraces me.

At my next physical therapy session, I don't need to say a word to my therapist. She can see all too clearly by the way I use both crutches, and grimace in pain. She suggests I have the doctor x-ray my left hip and leg at my follow up visit, but quickly reassures me this is only a precautionary measure.

"I don't expect the x-rays to show anything unusual," she adds in the kindest of voices.

I nod in agreement, but leave for home feeling frightened, and not in the least reassured.

The appointment with my doctor is scheduled for Tuesday, March 12th. I spend a sleepless night tossing and turning, trying to allay my fears. I feel in my bones something is terribly wrong, but have no idea as to what it might be. My doctor listens to my concerns and is supportive. She walks me to the x-ray technician, who helps me onto the table. A series of x-rays are quickly taken of my left and right hips and legs. Back in the examination room I sit for what feels like hours, watching the minutes tick by on the clock, as I wait for the x-rays to be read. Finally, the door opens and my doctor enters, a smile lighting her face.

"The x-rays appear normal," she says. "Everything seems to be fine."

I let out my breath, and silently offer a prayer of thanks. There is nothing seriously wrong with me after all.

CHAPTER 2

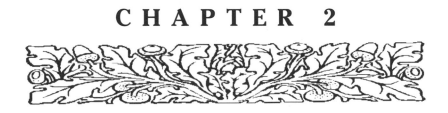

First, the Bad News

Sometimes, all it takes is a phone call to turn your life inside out, hurling you into a nightmare that until that very moment bears no relationship to reality as you know it. The call is from my doctor, and the news is not welcome. Upon further viewing, the x-rays show an ill defined lesion in the ball joint of my left hip. Both my doctor and the radiologist, who reread the x-ray, want me to have blood tests and a bone scan to rule out tumor, infection, or multiple myeloma which I am told is a form of cancer of the white blood cells. I am speechless and disbelieving. This cannot be happening to me. I try hard not to collapse into the overpowering wave of terror that spreads through my body. I remind myself that there are many possible explanations. Perhaps the lesion is scar tissue from an old birth injury. The main thing is to not panic.

I dread telling Stan, for he has been widowed only a little over a year. His wife Lynne, who he dearly loves, died in the company of family and friends, after a long and courageous battle with multiple sclerosis. Stan lives with his twenty one year old, broken hearted daughter Natalie, in the family home. He is still in the process of healing, and I don't know how he will handle my news. If he is the man I believe him to be, I feel he will continue to be there for me. My son Brent, and Stan's son Ari have been best friends since first grade, and we have known one another casually for many years through our children. I visited with Lynne during her illness, and Brent and I attended her funeral. I never thought of Stan as anything other than Ari and Natalie's father. I did not expect we would develop a close friendship, nor that it would grow into such a special relationship. I am grateful to have Stan in my life, and I am clear in wanting him to remain. When I tell Stan about the call, he is calm, loving and supportive. His strength is a blessing that I can count on.

I make a decision to not share this news with my children until I know something more conclusive. My reasoning is, if it turns out to be nothing, why upset them needlessly. And, if God forbid, it is a serious problem, that will be the time to let them know. In retrospect, I would not make this same decision. I would allow my children to be a part of the process from the beginning. We are family, and family sticks together through both the good and bad times. This is an important lesson my children have taught me, and it is one I have learned well.

That night I turn in prayer to God, asking God's help and protection. I affirm how very much I want to live. When I die, I want to be a wise, feisty old woman, who has lived through all the seasons of her life. I want to have done everything I deem important, and leave with no regrets.

"Please God," I pray, "grant me life. There is so much more I long to do and experience. I have little fear of death, but I am not ready to leave. I want to live to someday see my children have children of their own. I want to know the blessings of being a grandmother and great grandmother. I want years in which to weave the tapestry of my life in vibrant colors, and have my relationship with Stan shine brightly throughout it."

I fall asleep with the image in my mind of it all working out somehow.

The day I go for testing dawns cold and gray. I linger over my morning coffee, aware of my reluctance to leave for the hospital. I have never been overly fond of hospitals, and today I feel an overwhelming urge to escape to the warmth and sun of some tropical paradise. I promise myself that when this is all behind me, that is exactly what I will do. I leave with Stan, carrying two crystals in a small pouch, rose quartz for love and self healing, and amazonite for courage. Only later do I find out that Stan has even a more difficult time with hospitals than I do.

The testing is everything I fear it will be, cold, impersonal, and frightening. I must lay very still, not moving a muscle, while an unfamiliar machine slowly scans my body from head to toe. After awhile the technician returns with the results.

"There are two hot spots on your ribs, and one on your left hip. We need to take some chest x rays," she says.

"What are hot spots?" I ask with trepidation.

"Your doctor will talk to you about it," she answers, walking out of the room.

I return home hours later, feeling dehumanized, confused and very afraid.

Today is the first day of spring, a time for new life and new beginnings. How ironic that today I receive the test results. The news does not support the life force. The facts sound ominous. The chest x-ray shows a mass at the top of my left lung. The unofficial diagnosis is lung cancer, that has metastasized to my hip and ribs. I don't believe it. I stopped smoking over ten years ago. There must be some mistake. I wonder if this is what is meant by shock and denial. I want to bargain, to promise anything. Just make it not be true. I remember Stan saying the other day, that you always have to have your bags packed. My bags may be packed, but I am not ready to go.

I am unable to contain myself when Stan comes by, and begin sobbing immediately.

"What's wrong Susan? Tell me. Tell me." Stan keeps repeating.

All I can sob over and over is, "I don't want to tell you. I don't want you to know."

Stan leads me to the couch, and holds me for a very long time. I calm down enough to blurt out the nightmare.

"I don't want to do this to you," I say. "You just lost Lynne a little over a year ago."

A YEAR OF MIRACLES

"You have to let me love you," Stan insists. "Me, and all the people who love you. You have to receive our love, Susan. I was there for Lynne, and I want to be there for you."

"You loved Lynne, and were committed to her," I reply. "She was your wife, but it's different between us. I know how much you care about me, but you aren't committed to me. You can't even tell me you love me, because I love you means a lifelong commitment to you." I fall silent for a moment and then continue. "Even though you can't say it to me, I can say it to you because I do love you, and it doesn't have to mean marriage and forevermore."

Stan looks into my eyes and there are tears in his. "I do love you Susan, and it is the purest of loves. It doesn't have to come from commitment or marriage. The time we have is indefinite. We don't know how long it will be, but we will go through it together, and we will make it wonderful," he says in a voice trembling with emotion.

Tears fill my eyes, and spill over. I am crying a lot today. "I am glad, I am so glad," I keep repeating.

I rest in Stan's arms, as he holds me. This is the man I have waited for my entire life. I want years and years with him. Lifetimes. I am not willing to die. I will heal from this cancer, if that is what it truly is. I will do all in my power to live. I love life. I am going to live. That's all there is to it. People can heal from cancer. People can even heal from metastasized cancer. Stan's father-in-law had colon cancer that metastasized to his liver. Ten years later, he is alive, active, and healthy. It has been ten years since my dear friend Susan healed from breast cancer. We call ourselves the Brooklyn Babes, and share such a deep and loving bond. Now we will share this challenge as well. My client Jackie had advanced lung cancer five years ago. I worked with her, and helped her heal. I believe I too can heal from cancer, especially with so very much to live for.

Stan wants to spend the night, but despite his desire to, he has to return home. His body has become both chilled and numb. He is visibly shivering, and feels physically exhausted. Stan says this is how his body responds to shock and trauma. It shuts down, forcing him to sleep so it can repair itself. He says it would be a comfort to stay with me, but he doesn't feel that he can. As much as I would like him to remain, I know we both need some time alone tonight. Besides, there is a phone call I still have to make.

I dial Marilyn's number in California, knowing the unbearable pain my words will bring into her life. We are the dearest of friends, and call ourselves "soul sisters and keepers of the sacred flame." We can, and do, finish each others sentences. We know what the other is thinking and feeling without the need for words. We share almost twenty years of memories, adventures, spirituality, love, laughter, and tears. Though we now live thousands of miles apart, our bond only grows stronger. We often joke that the money we spend staying in touch keeps the phone company and airlines solvent, and there is some truth to that. As I expect, I can feel my news shattering Marilyn. She tries hard to be strong and comfort me, as I do her, but we both break down and sob uncontrollably. To comfort one another tonight is an impossibility.

Marilyn promises to obtain an immediate reading with Michael, who is a channel, in order to gain additional spiritual insight into the cancer diagnosis and the root causes behind it. What Michael does is enter a deep meditative trance, where he receives messages about the person in question. Michael believes that the messages come from the spiritual realm, bringing pertinent information that is important to that person's well being. I readily agree to the reading. I have had readings that I have found helpful in the past. I am open to anything that can enlighten me, and may help me heal.

Before attempting to sleep, there is one more thing I must do. I enter into a meditative state, ask God to show me why this is happening now, and draw a Rune. The Rune I draw is Wholeness. This Rune speaks of the impulse towards self-realization and regeneration, the letting of the Light into a part of life that has been secret or shut away, and the profound recognition of what has long been denied in order to accomplish this. I replace the Rune, vigorously shake the bag to mix the Runes, and ask a final question.

"God," I pray, "what will be the final outcome?"

Once again, I draw the Rune of Wholeness. As I do, a sense of peacefulness, hope, and expectancy sustains me. I know that with help from God, I will be able to let the Light into the secret and hidden part of my life. I fall asleep, comforted by the knowledge that my healing partnership with God has already begun.

CHAPTER 3

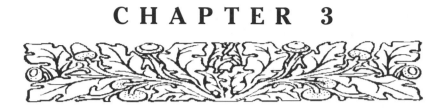

Reaching Out

Marilyn calls to say the tape of Michael's channeling is in the mail, along with additional healing and meditation tapes. But there is information she wants to share with me now. According to Michael, the emotional component of cancer is anger. Deep hurt. Long-standing resentment. All cause an eating away at the self. This is not news to me. I have heard and read this before. What is news, and shocking, is that Michael sees hidden secret pockets of resentment, hurt, and anger running through me. He spells them out. It is up to me he says. This is a wake up call. My will to live is extremely significant. If I work toward releasing the areas he has outlined, there can be a miraculous healing. It is up to me, he repeats. Not just me, I think. It is up to God and me. We are partners.

I place a call to Gwen, my friend and teacher whom I dearly love. Gwen has worked as a licensed psychologist for many years, but now spends her time conducting workshops in Sacred Psychology throughout the United States and Canada. She is a gifted healer, very psychic, and I trust her insights. Gwen immediately states that she does not see me dying.

"I see a fight on your hands. A battle. A clenched jaw and fist. Determination. Not an angry fight. Rather a fight of strength. A test. A hard, hard test. A trial by fire. Fire to burn away the extraneous. A transformation and discovery of your True Self. Speak and act lovingly to your body," she advises me. "It needs all the support it can get. Make love. Help heal your body through sex."

A YEAR OF MIRACLES

I laugh when she says this, knowing I have a very willing partner.

"This is an incredibly exciting time for you," Gwen continues. "Something wonderful is going to happen with Susan. It flies in the face of all we know now. It might even look worse before it gets better, but it will get better. Let go of your angers, resentments and old hurts. Release them. It is time to let others off the hook for injuries they have caused you in the past. Shed, release and cleanse. Forgive them."

I can feel Gwen's love and her confidence in my healing across the many miles that separate us. She promises to hold me cradled in her heart, and do many healings and meditations on my behalf. Feeling blessed, nurtured, and comforted, I say my good-byes.

Much of the day is spent meditating and reflecting on the messages from Gwen and Michael. They are crystal clear. It is up to me to acknowledge, forgive and release those persons and situations towards whom I hold suppressed anger, resentment and hurt. It is as the Rune of Wholeness says, letting the Light into a part of my life that has been secret and shut away. To accomplish this requires a profound recognition of what until now I have denied, the hidden angers, hurts and resentments. I make a crucial decision. I will do whatever it takes to heal. I will open to these feelings, and allow the Light to cleanse and heal this suppressed negativity. I will embrace forgiveness whole heartedly. I will make whatever amends I can. I will, with the help of God, family, friends, and the traditional and alternative healing communities, move toward wholeness and healing.

That night I have a significant dream. I am being chased by a dark figure I cannot see. I know pure terror. My heart pounds, as adrenaline courses throughout my body. The lump in my throat barely allows me to swallow, my stomach is twisted in knots, and my breathing is labored. Time and again, I just manage to escape whatever is chasing me. Suddenly the scene changes and I find myself in a room. It is large, airy, and painted white, with a wall of floor to ceiling windows overlooking a serene landscape of rolling green hills, large blooming trees, and a profusion of brightly colored flowers. On each side of the main window are two smaller windows that lock in the center. I run to the windows on the left, then to the windows on the right, and lock them. The locks are as clear as the glass. Looking outside at the breathtaking view, the dark figure is nowhere in sight. The terror subsides and I feel safe. I awaken from the dream knowing the figure chasing me is my shadow side, the hidden part of me I refuse to face.

I recognize this dream as delivering a timely message, which I accept as a gift. I cannot run away from my fears, my angers, my resentments, my demons, my hurts. I have to bring them to light, face and vanquish them. I must become a spiritual warrior, one whose battle is always with the self. Otherwise, I will remain imprisoned, looking out at the beauty and richness of life, but separated from experiencing it fully and freely, by an invisible barrier of my own making.

I am reading from a book of spiritual writings, and meditating on the words, "I will to will Thy will." I think about how difficult those words could be to truly live out, for if God's Will were for me to die, I would not want to will it. I open my eyes and, for the briefest of moments, see a flash of light upon the wall, and simultaneously receive a message that says, "My will is for you to live." Tears flood my eyes, and gratitude fills my heart, for I know that in willing to will God's Will, I am willing the life force. The remainder of the day, I feel peaceful, centered and serene. I am aware of what I need to do, and feel confident in my ability to succeed, but most importantly, I know God is on my side.

A YEAR OF MIRACLES

CHAPTER 4

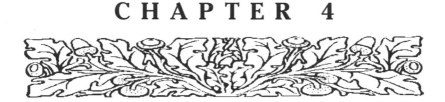

Diagnosis

I awaken to a beautiful, sunny spring day. It is a fitting day to celebrate the twenty seventh birthday of my daughter Sharon. As I reflect upon her birth, I marvel once again, how swiftly time passes. It seems just a heartbeat ago, I held my firstborn in my arms, and felt such a powerful surge of love for this new and precious life entrusted to my care. That love has only grown deeper and stronger with the passage of years. I have been truly blessed to have had that experience two additional times, with the subsequent births of my daughter Elyssa, and my son Brent. It is important to hold the specialness of today in my heart, for I will be undergoing my first CAT scan this evening, and I am frightened of what it may reveal.

Susan comes with me for the scan, and I find her presence comforting. Having walked a similar path in overcoming cancer, she is completely in tune with what I am feeling. She talks with me for hours on end, about her own fears, hopes, mindset, and eventual triumph. Susan reminds me she is only doing what I did for her ten years ago. She is like a beacon of light, steady and strong, helping me see the way. Her faith in God and in my healing are unshakable. Is it any wonder I love Susan, and think of her as the sister I never had? Add to that, the offbeat east coast humor we inspire in one another, our shared dreams, joys, and sorrows, oddly similar backgrounds as "Jewish Brooklyn Babes," a strong spiritual-emotional bonding, plus fifteen years of "being family,"… and a picture of the depth and breadth of our relationship begins to emerge.

A YEAR OF MIRACLES

Despite my desire to be otherwise, I feel scared and vulnerable lying on a cold metal table, trying to visualize a healthy body free of disease, surrounded by white light. My imaging continuously gets disrupted as the technician keeps repeating in a monotone, "Take a deep breath. Hold it. Breathe," while the noisy machine above me, takes picture after picture. There are tears in my eyes, and I find it hard to retain my courage. These past two weeks are taking a heavy emotional toll, and all the love, support and nurturance cannot completely eradicate the terror that lies just under the surface, waiting for an opportunity to erupt. Right now, although I know better, God feels very far away.

Hours later, following a long sob and hot bubble bath that helps ease some of my fears, I write the following in my journal.

> "When this is all behind me and I find myself blessed with good health and wholeness, I will share this journey with others, to help nurture them and offer hope. I will write a book about my experience with cancer and how I healed. I will work with others with life threatening illnesses, doing all I can to help them heal. I will continue deepening my spiritual partnership with God, by developing ever increasing faith and trust that God is Goodness, Divine Order, Love and Light. I will do whatever I can to help make the world a better place, and have my life make a difference. And every day from the depths of my being, I will praise God and give thanks for my healing. This I promise. This promise I will keep."

At 3:00 a.m. Elyssa calls, apologetic, but urgently needing to talk. Unable to sleep because of a major career decision she has to make by morning, she is anxious and stressed. At 23, Elyssa is trying to decide between the safety and security of the known, and the risk and promise of the unknown. After a lengthy conversation, it becomes clear that despite the risks involved, Elyssa wants to make the change. I am proud of my daughter for not letting fear deter her from moving forward in life. Like mother, like daughter, I think dreamily, drifting back to sleep.

I am angry upon rising, and as the day progresses my anger burns brighter. Aware that the suppressed angers, hurts, and resentments of the past are surfacing, and that it is time to begin releasing them, I borrow Brent's paddleball racket and, using both crutches, slowly navigate into the bedroom. Kneeling beside the bed, I raise the racket high over my head, striking the mattress again and again, as low guttural sounds erupt from my throat. My voice gets louder and shriller, until I am yelling and raging at the top of my lungs. I feel the anger like steam, rise up from hidden recesses of my being. Mocha, my beloved eleven year old Golden Retriever/Samoyed rushes into the room barking in alarm. I motion for her to leave, and she retreats to just outside the door, where she settles uneasily, keeping me in clear sight. Crouched and covered in sweat, I am in an absolute frenzy, unable to recall half of what I am raging about. Perhaps the words I utter don't really matter, for as I continue to discharge, I find myself breathing more deeply and fully, knowing a healing of both body and soul is occurring.

As I fall silent, Mocha cautiously re-enters the room, walks to my side, and begins licking the tears from my face. We sit together for the longest of time, my arms wrapped around Mocha's neck, her tail wagging fiercely, two old friends giving and receiving comfort. I can sense a difference inside me. A letting go of darkness. An opening to Light. At this moment, I have total trust I will emerge from this journey whole and healed.

Stan and I go out to dinner and a movie. For a few precious hours, we are just two people enjoying time spent together. Laughing. Loving. Having fun. We return home to a phone call from my doctor that instantly changes that. The report on the CAT scan does not show lung cancer, but there is no reason to rejoice. Instead, it shows a large mass in the lower abdomen and two suspicious areas in the liver. The unofficial diagnosis is kidney cancer which has metastasized to the left hip, my second and seventh ribs, and most likely to my liver. A rib biopsy has been scheduled to confirm the newest diagnosis. This is the first time I have been told point blank that I have cancer, and a wave of fear floods through every part of my body. No cancer is ever desirable, but I know metastasized kidney cancer is a particularly dismal one to heal from, for the standard medical treatments of surgery, radiation and chemotherapy are highly ineffective. Stan's immediate reaction is to become very angry at the way I am being treated. He likens it to being in an automobile repair shop, where the diagnosis of the problem keeps changing. There is safety for Stan in feeling anger instead of fear, so for tonight his anger comforts him.

My ex-husband Norm makes inquiries on my behalf. He is a full professor at the College of Pharmacy, at The University of Michigan. Over the years, Norm has received many research grants from the National Institutes of Health and numerous prestigious institutions. Norm is well positioned in the scientific community, and knows many leading physicians and researchers throughout the world. He has found out that experimental immunotherapy is being used to treat advanced kidney cancer at the National Institutes of Health. Norm has spoken with Dr. Steven Rosenberg, who pioneered this treatment, and Dr. Rosenberg is willing to see and evaluate me as a candidate for his program. Norm learns that Dr. Alfred Chang, who worked with Dr. Rosenberg on this protocol at the National Institutes of Health, is currently involved in researching the use of experimental immunotherapy on advanced kidney cancer patients at the University of Michigan Medical Center. It is one of only four or five such programs in the country, and it is in my hometown of Ann Arbor. I am grateful to learn there is a new promising medical treatment available, and that it is available here.

Norm agrees that it is time I talk to our children. He assures me he will do all in his power to help them through this difficult time. I am especially thankful Norm and I have the warm, caring friendship we do. I need all the support I can get, and knowing my children will be able to turn to their father is a great help. I need to believe I will ultimately emerge victorious, but what a challenge of faith this is right now.

Sharon stops by in the early afternoon, after her last class at the University of Michigan School of Social Work, where she is enrolled for her Masters in Social Work. She can tell as soon as she sees me, something is terribly wrong. As I relay the news, the color drains from her face and she begins to tremble.

"Mom, I don't think I can deal with this," she says in a voice wracked with pain.

"Sharon," I say tears rolling down my cheeks, "you don't have a choice. You have to."

We hug. We kiss. We cry together. I promise Sharon I will fight to live. I tell her I need her love, support, strength and belief in me. She unhesitatingly responds that I have it unconditionally, and insists on going with me for the rib biopsy the following day. Sharon wants to be there in whatever way she can. I feel confident Sharon will find the courage and strength to deal with this crisis and emerge the stronger for it. I am especially grateful she has the love and support of her husband Chuck to help her through this. He is a good man, strong, steady, calm, and nurturing.

It is not any easier telling Elyssa. She is also visibly effected, and I see fear spring to life in her eyes.

"I dreamt I had cancer just a few nights ago," Elyssa says between sobs. "It must have been a premonition about you mom."

"I'm glad it's not you," I truthfully answer. "Your life is just beginning. If it has to be one of us, I'd rather it be me."

Once again, I voice my need for Elyssa's love, strength, support and belief in my ability to heal. She offers it without hesitation. I know intuitively Elyssa will be able to weather this difficult time, for she has all the inner and outer resources necessary to do so.

A YEAR OF MIRACLES

I decide to tell Brent over the weekend. He is a sophomore at the University of Michigan, and has two major exams within the next two days. I have waited this long. I can wait a little longer. I insist Sharon and Elyssa not talk with Brent until after I do, and they agree. I do not know it then, but I will not have the opportunity to tell Brent in the way I am so carefully planning.

There are two more of "my children" I still need to speak to. Tracy and Jennifer are not my biological children, but they are children of my heart. Elyssa and Jennifer have been inseparable friends since third grade, and Jennifer becomes one of the family, and another one of my children. At sixteen, Jennifer loses her beloved mother Marilyn to cancer. On her deathbed, Marilyn requests that I care for Jennifer as if she were my own daughter. I immediately promise to do so, and I have not regretted making or keeping that promise.

Tracy enters my life shortly before her sixth birthday, when her father and I become romantically involved in a relationship that lasts over four years. During most of that time, Tracy, her father, Sharon, Elyssa, Brent and I live together as a family. In the ensuing years we maintain an ongoing contact. When she turns fifteen, seemingly insurmountable problems arise between Tracy and her father, and she comes to live with our family. Three years later, Musical Theater Scholarship in hand, Tracy leaves for college and a dormitory room at the University of Michigan School of Music. Though she is reunited with her father, Tracy frequently returns home for holidays, visits, winter and spring breaks, and all major family occasions. She is truly one of my children.

I am emotionally spent from talking with Sharon and Elyssa, and decide to talk to both Tracy and Jennifer sometime over the weekend. As with Brent, this will not work out the way I am planning.

CHAPTER 5

Misdiagnosis

I experience both apprehension and excitement the morning of the rib biopsy. Apprehension over possibly learning I have kidney cancer. Excitement, because I am planning to raise my consciousness outside of my physical body. I will be doing this to avoid experiencing the excruciating pain involved in this procedure, for which no anesthetic can be given. I have done this in the past, but never under such trying circumstances. In a reality that has been feeling out of control lately, this is one area in which I am able to exert a small measure of control. Sharon and Susan accompany me to the hospital. To a casual observer it would appear we are in a festive mood, for the joking and laughter we engage in, masks our mutual anxiety.

I change into a hospital gown that ties down the back, and then enter a sterile white room, filled with large pieces of machinery and bright overhead lights. I am told to climb onto the table and lie on my stomach. Holding a piece of selenite for raised consciousness in one hand and an amethyst crystal for a meditative visionary state in the other, I position myself on the table. An area of my back is exposed, scrubbed, and painted. I am swathed in many gauzelike pieces of fabric and must lie absolutely still. I feel like I am in the center of a cocoon, where I only hear voices, but see no one. Perhaps I will emerge a butterfly I dreamily think.

The doctor lets me know each time he is about to insert the needle into my second rib. I begin raising my consciousness, by closing my eyes, and breathing deeply and rhythmically. I can feel the energy at the base of my spine slowly travel upwards to the top of my head, and then through it. I experience this energy as hovering about six inches above my crown. In this altered state, I do not feel the needle enter my second rib, and am only vaguely aware of what is happening around me.

Instead, I find myself floating in a peaceful, safe, secure space. I am in the center of a circle that has no beginning or end, and I am surrounded by Stan, my children, my family and friends. My mother and grandmother though both deceased, are also with me. Further out in the circle are people I know on a more casual basis. Beyond them are many more people I don't recognize at all. All of the people in the circle are smiling, and are sending healing energy toward me. I can feel the healing energies as they enter and vibrate throughout my whole body. I close my eyes and bask in the warmth and love of the healing circle.

When next I open my eyes, a wedding is taking place. I recognize that the bride and groom are Stan and myself. We are radiant, in excellent health, head over heels in love and beaming with joy. Once again we are surrounded by loving family and friends. They are toasting us and calling out "mazel tov" (happiness) and "l'chaim" (to life). Though we have no plans to marry, and what I have seen is only a vision, a wedding much like this one will unite us in marriage, fifteen months from now on July 12, 1992.

Upon returning to the outpatient recovery room, Sharon and Susan are waiting in the cubicle that will become home for the next two hours. I share both visions with them and we unanimously agree that I will only tell Stan about the healing circle. After all, why inform him about our wedding before he has even decided he wants to marry me? It is enough that I know for now. He will find out soon enough.

A young nurse who is monitoring my vital signs, brings in three glasses of orange juice and joins in our conversation.
"What are you here for," she asks?

"I've just had a rib biopsy, and am waiting for the results, which will show if I have kidney cancer," I tell her. "There is a possibility that it may be multiple myeloma. At least that's what the doctors say."

"It would be preferable if it were multiple myeloma," she responds. "It is a slow growing cancer, and you can live with it for upwards of twenty years or more."

"I don't want to have either, but if I have to have cancer, my choice is multiple myeloma," I answer.

"Me too," says Sharon.

"Me three," says Susan.

"Me four," adds my nurse with a smile.

A feeling of mutual camaraderie in a little cubicle of a large and largely impersonal medical center is firmly established amongst the four of us.

The doctor who performed the rib biopsy enters the cubicle looking grim.

"I am sorry to have to tell you this, but you do have cancer," he says gently. "The biopsy shows you have multiple myeloma."

"That's great," I say overjoyed. "That's really good news. Thank you."

A smile spreads across my face.

Susan and Sharon let out a loud Brooklyn cheer. My new friend the nurse winks at me and smiles broadly. The doctor's face mirrors his confusion.

"You are the very first patient I have met who is actually happy to learn she has cancer," he says sounding puzzled. "Why is that?"

"Please don't think that I'm crazy," I reply. "Though I would understand if you do. It's not that I'm pleased to have cancer. I could have lived my whole life happily without cancer, and never missed the experience. It's just that I was afraid the rib biopsy would show I had advanced kidney cancer, which I know has a very dismal prognosis."

"I understand your happiness now," he responds, the confusion fading from his face. "You are a brave and courageous woman. I am very impressed with how you dealt with the rib biopsy. I believe you will do well, for you possess the qualities of a cancer survivor."

I smile broadly, and reach out to shake his hand.

"I completely agree with you," I reply honestly. "I plan to heal from cancer, and live a long and happy life."

Suddenly I am ravenously hungry, and Sharon and Susan head to the cafeteria for food and drinks. Upon returning, we toast in celebration of my latest diagnosis. It feels very strange to actually be celebrating a diagnosis of cancer, and the irony does not escape us.

"We're just three weird wacky women," we joke, as once again we toast to the "good news" of multiple myeloma.

Later that evening Stan and I reenact a similar ritual, by going out to dinner and celebrating my diagnosis. Still, in the back of my mind there is a nagging voice I try hard to ignore, but cannot.

"You have been misdiagnosed before," it whispers. "What makes you so certain, that you haven't been misdiagnosed once again?"

CHAPTER 6

Emergency and Re-diagnosis

Although I am not religious in a traditional sense, Passover is a Jewish Holiday I enjoy celebrating. From the time I attend my first Passover Seder at Great Aunt Anna's house, where as the youngest child I have the honor of asking the four questions, Passover holds a special place in my heart. Despite the fact that I am facing a serious health crisis, I find myself singing as I get ready for tonight's Seder. My good friend and business partner Pat will be bringing me to the Seder, for I am no longer able to drive. The Seder will be an opportunity to share with a loving and caring group of friends the challenge I am facing, and ask for their prayers and support.

This year, for the first time, the Seder will not be held at June's house, and that saddens me. Pat, June, and I, have been the closest of friends, as well as business partners for over fifteen years at Tapestry, the counseling center we founded. Using massive doses of humor and laughter in our daily interactions has helped us to diffuse a potential "burn out" profession. Pat and I are still adjusting to June's recent move to California. Despite speaking with June often, I miss her, and wish she were here tonight. It is hard to lose one of the "Three Musketeers," as we call ourselves, and not feel at least a little off center. Especially when the missing musketeer is the one who insists on being in the center of every picture taken of the three of us.

A YEAR OF MIRACLES

The Seder goes as I have envisioned. My friends are encouraging, and rally around me. I feel their love and concern. I will come through this whole I promise them. Next year the Seder will be at my house. We raise glasses and toast to this promise. Later, reading from the Passover Hagaddah about how the homes of the Jews were marked and the Angel of Death passed over them, I make a silent prayer.

"Please God, may the Angel of Death pass over me as well."

After a long, gratifying evening, Pat and I say our good-byes and leave. As I walk down the front step, an excruciating pain shoots up my left hip and leg, rendering me immobile. My leg refuses to work, and any attempt on my part to use it is torturous. Bathed in agony, I vaguely perceive a group of ashen faced friends gathered around me. Despite their urging, I refuse to allow anyone to call an ambulance. I am insistent upon going home. I know this is irrational behavior on my part, but I am past caring. I can't bear the thought of ending up in the emergency room in the middle of the night. I want some control over my destiny, and one more night in my own bed. Pat and June's brother Gary half drag, half carry me into the car, then into my house, and finally onto my waterbed.

"I'll do anything for attention," I half heartedly attempt to joke, but one look at Pat and Gary's grim faces and I fall silent.

It is decided that Pat will spend the night with me. She brings a pillow and blanket into my room, and hastily assembles a makeshift bed on the floor. As long as I don't move, I don't hurt. But the slightest movement is unbearable and brings tears to my eyes. When I need to use the toilet, Pat has to slide a plastic container under me. The process is slow and painful, and that night I learn the true meaning of bladder control. Neither Pat's or my own feeble attempts at humor work. We are both too frightened to pretend otherwise. Still, having Pat glued to my side throughout that excruciatingly long night makes it much easier to bear. She is truly a Godsend.

EMERGENCY AND RE-DIAGNOSIS

At the first light of dawn, I phone my doctor at her home and explain the situation. It is obvious to both of us that there is no way I can come to her office.

"Call an ambulance immediately," she unequivocally states. "You must go to the hospital now. I will alert them, so that they will expect you."

I hang up the phone and turn to Pat, tears in my eyes.

"She want's me to go to the hospital right away," I say.

"Good idea," says Pat. "So do I."

"It's just that you don't like bedpan duty," I reply tearfully.

"Right," Pat answers, and gently hugs me.

Before calling for an ambulance, I dial Sharon's number. She answers and I tell her what has taken place.

"I'm on my way," she replies in a strained voice. "I want to ride to the hospital with you. I'll call the ambulance when I get there."

I dial Elyssa's house, but get no answer. Later, I will learn she is out running. I decide against calling Stan, as I recall the difficulty he has with hospitals. I can spare him for the moment, although he will find out soon enough. Sharon arrives looking distraught, and quickly dials 911. In only minutes the ambulance arrives, and my bedroom fills with paramedics, trying to figure out how to lift me onto the stretcher.

While they confer, the phone rings and I automatically answer it. My heart sinks when I hear Brent's voice. This is not how I want to tell my son, but I have no choice but to do so now. I hear a sharp intake of breath as I speak, and when Brent responds his voice is taut and shaking.

"I'll meet you in the emergency room, mom."

I begin to cry. "I'm so sorry Brent. I didn't want you to find out this way. I was going to tell you this weekend."

"It's okay mom. Really. Don't worry about it now."

A young paramedic taps me on the shoulder. "Ma'am, we're going to try lifting you now."

"Brent, I have to get off the phone. They're about ready to take me to the hospital," I say.

"Okay mom, I'm on my way there."

"I love you Brent."

"Same here mom."

I slowly hang up the phone, and dab at the tears on my face. Sharon hands me some Kleenex.

"Sharon, please make sure that Tracy and Jennifer know," I say as the paramedics converge at my bedside. "I was going to tell them this weekend."

"I'll take care of it," she promises. "Consider it done."

Every time the paramedics attempt to lift me out of the waterbed, I howl in pain. Finally, they arrive at a solution. Lifting up the waterbed sheet with me on it, they carry me to the waiting ambulance. I scream and scream. I cannot bear the pain.

"Give her a shot of something strong," I hear Sharon yelling at them. "My mother is in agony."

I feel a needle enter my vein, and mercifully the pain starts receding.

"What about me?" Sharon sobs, tears streaming down her face. "Can you give me something to ease my pain?"

I hang onto Sharon's hand, drifting in and out of consciousness as the sirens scream and the ambulance races to the emergency room at the University of Michigan Medical Center.

I remember only bits and pieces over the next few days, for I am heavily medicated for the excruciating pain of what turns out to be a broken hip. I am vaguely aware of being taken for another rib biopsy, x-rays and a full body scan, but mostly I am disoriented and groggy when awake. Stan, Susan, and my children are constantly by my side. Pat and other friends drift in and out. Marilyn calls two and three times a day, although I have no recollection of our conversations. The orthopedic surgeon catches me at one of my more lucid moments, and informs me that I will be undergoing surgery for a hip joint replacement Tuesday morning. I just passively nod in agreement, and ask no questions. I don't want to hear any answers.

I am told the surgery goes very well, that the orthopedic surgeon who performs it is one of the best in the field. With

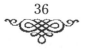

physical and occupational therapy I should make a full recovery within a couple of months. A few days later, I begin physical and occupational therapy. Among other things, I learn how to walk up and down steps, get in and out of a car, dress myself, and put on and take off my shoes.

I learn what has caused my hip to break when the orthopedic surgeon enters my room, flanked by physicians, residents, interns, and medical students. He stands as far away from my bed as possible, and avoids looking at me, as he delivers his news.

"Your hip is healing nicely," he begins. "However, there is a more serious problem. Our laboratory tests show dead cancer cells in your hip. It was cancer that ate through your hip and caused it to break. Since there is nothing more I can do for you, we will be moving you upstairs to the oncology unit later today. Good luck."

As he finishes speaking, he turns his back on me, and followed by his entourage beats a hasty retreat.

Stan and I stare at one another speechless. I am stunned. Much later, after processing my anger towards this incredibly insensitive man, I will nickname him Dr. Compassion, but at the time all I feel is total devastation and pure unadulterated terror. It will be a year before Stan shares with me what he has overheard in the corridor outside my room, just before Dr. Compassion makes his grand entrance.

Hearing voices in the hallway, Stan moves to the door, while oblivious to the voices, I continue leafing through a magazine.

"Have you heard the one about the doctor and the patient?" chuckles Dr. Compassion to the assembled physicians on rounds.

"The good news, Mr. Jones, is that the lab report says you have a month to live."

"Doctor, if that's the good news, what can possibly be worse than that?"

"The bad news, Mr. Jones, is that I was on vacation for three weeks when the lab report came in."

A YEAR OF MIRACLES

"The good news for this patient is that the hip joint replacement was a complete success. The bad news is that it doesn't make a difference, because she is terminally ill with advanced metastasized kidney cancer," Dr. Compassion pronounces, as he enters my room.

CHAPTER 7

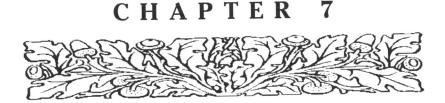

Angels of Darkness, Angels of Light

The assault on my senses continues throughout the day. Reeling from the news I have just heard, I seek comfort from Stan, and minutes later from Sharon, who has just entered the room. Despite their own shock and pain, they give to me unfailingly, reassuring me that I will survive this nightmare and emerge whole. As our voices fall silent, we join hands and pray, asking God to bestow Tender Mercies on me. Stan, visibly aging within the span of an hour, promises to return quickly, and rushes out to purchase the three books I have requested. They are "Getting Well Again," by O. Carl Simonton M.D. and Stephanie Simonton, "Love, Medicine and Miracles," and "Peace, Love and Healing," both by Dr. Bernie Siegel. They are to become a lifeline in the months to follow.

Only minutes later the door opens, and the head floor nurse enters my room with unwelcome information.

"You will be transferred to the oncology floor later this afternoon," she says.

"I am not going to move," I say forcefully. "You can have this room when I am discharged."

Staring at me as if I am slightly demented, and ignoring my response to her news, she continues talking about the impending move.

"Listen to me," I finally say in exasperation. "I told you I wasn't changing rooms. I meant it."

Clearly, this nurse is at a loss as to a response. I am not following hospital rules and playing my role of good patient.

A YEAR OF MIRACLES

I am both a troublemaker and a bad patient, and she is not used to dealing with patients like me.

"You will have to speak with my supervisor," she responds and flees the room.

Sharon and I look at one another, and burst out laughing. The laughter temporarily disperses the tension and fear that cling to us, and comes as a welcome relief.

"You are one tough woman," Sharon says admiringly. "Don't let anyone mess with my mom."

"You've got that right," I agree. "Watch out world. Here I come."

In a relatively short time, the dispute is resolved. I will remain in my present room until I am discharged. I am viewed as stubborn and uncooperative, but I don't mind. It feels empowering to be able to exercise some small measure of control over my life today. Later, I will read in one of Dr. Siegel's books, that assertive, appropriately non compliant patients who question the voice of authority, generally fare better and outlive the passive, don't cause trouble good patients, hospitals seem to so dearly love.

A young, attractive woman wearing a white lab coat, quietly slips into the room. It takes a moment for me to realize she is a doctor, because of her extremely youthful appearance.

"I've come to speak with you because you have kidney cancer," she says, sadness etched on her face, "and I have a special interest in your particular kind of cancer."

"What do you mean kidney cancer?" I ask startled. "I was diagnosed with multiple myeloma."

"The diagnosis was wrong. It is definitely kidney cancer," answers the voice of authority. "We did a full body scan on you earlier this week, and it clearly shows a large mass on your left kidney. That is known as your primary tumor. The tumors on your ribs and liver are secondary ones, and have spread from the primary tumor. As for your hip, that is kidney cancer that has spread to the bone, and eaten it away."

"No," I moan. "It's not true. I don't believe you."

"Look," she says, "I can bring you the scan, and you can see it for yourself. Do you want me to?"

"Yes," I sob, and she turns to leave.

I glance over at Sharon. She is as white as a ghost, and she is shaking uncontrollably. I move over in bed, and Sharon crawls in besides me. We wrap our arms around each other in a tight embrace, and lying side by side surrender to our mutual grief.

There is something healing in the very act of releasing unbearable pain. Although the external circumstances may remain the same as before, there is a subtle yet perceptible inner shift that allows one to endure the unendurable. By the time the doctor returns with the printout of the scan, Sharon and I are ready. To my untrained eye, I cannot see the bulge that makes this doctor so certain I have kidney cancer, nor can Sharon. The doctor runs her finger over an area on the scan.

"This is it right here," she points.

I strain once again to see what she sees and fail.

"You could be wrong," I begin, desperately trying to find another explanation. "You just have a picture that makes you think so. The rib biopsy showed otherwise."

There is no doubt by the tone of her voice, that she is fast losing patience with me. She is the doctor. She is the expert. She is not used to having her knowledge questioned by a mere patient.

"We are still waiting for the results of the rib biopsy we did earlier this week," she admits. "However, we expect it to confirm a kidney cancer diagnosis. It is unfortunate you were misdiagnosed twice, but that sometimes happens. If I were you, I wouldn't get my hopes up."

"You aren't me," I angrily shoot back.

"Look," she says turning gentle. "You are terribly upset, and you don't want to accept what I am telling you, but it is the truth. I know a lot about kidney cancer. More than I would want to, really. My father died from kidney cancer, and since then I have specialized in it. I would like to be your primary physician as you go through the different stages of this disease."

Go through the stages I think, and suddenly I know with a certainty. A chill runs through my body as I look into her eyes. There is sadness in those eyes, but something else resides there and it is certain death. She has already written me off. Although I am still a vital, living, breathing human being, Dr. Death knows that I am going to die, just as her father did.

"I am planning on living, and I will find a doctor who believes that is possible. A doctor who will work toward helping me heal," I say with all the dignity I can muster. "I don't yet know who that doctor will be, but I do know it won't be you."

Startled by my outburst, Dr. Death looks at me, and for the first time since entering my room, really sees me. Without saying a word, she quickly crosses the room and with one backward, sorrowful glance, quietly closes the door. Sharon and I smile at each other, and silently embrace.

It takes awhile for my full anger at Dr. Death to surface, but when it does it bubbles over. Why I question, did she drop this bombshell on me late Friday afternoon, and then leave for the weekend? What was her point? Wouldn't it be more compassionate, and make more sense to wait until the results of the rib biopsy are known? Hospitals pretty much shut down for the weekend, except for emergencies, and I am no longer considered an immediate emergency. Why not wait until Monday, and then speak with me? At best this is extreme insensitivity, and an unthought out act of stupidity. Why the rush to inform me late Friday afternoon? The more I think about it, the angrier I feel myself becoming.

I decide to do a reality check in case I am over reacting. Given all that has happened today, I accept that as a real possibility. I talk with Stan, my children, Marilyn, Susan, and Pat. They are even angrier than I am. The consensus of opinion is the same. It is a totally uncalled for, and thoroughly unwarranted behavior on the doctor's part. To leave me hanging like this over the weekend is cruel. Armed with their indignation, which only feeds my own, I make a decision to do something about the situation. I call for the nurse, and when she enters, inform her I want to file a formal complaint about my treatment at the hands of Dr. Death. Hearing me out, she looks at me warily, but does not attempt to dissuade me. I suspect my reputation as a troublemaker is well known on the floor by now. She promises to note the complaint on my chart, and personally see that it finds its way to the Chief of Oncology.

"I appreciate your assistance," I say warmly. "I will be looking forward to a response. Thank you."

"You're welcome," she answers, as she vigorously plumps up my pillows.

I am reading "Getting Well Again," when Dr. Max Wicha enters my room. Although I do not know it at the time, I will later learn that he is Chief of the Division of Hematology and Oncology. I like Dr. Wicha from the start. There is an openness and warmth that he emanates, and when he speaks, he looks at me, and really sees me.

"I understand today has been a rough day for you," he begins. "I am sorry, and can only imagine how frightening this must be."

Tears fill my eyes. Finally. A doctor I can relate to.

"It's terrifying," I acknowledge, "And it's made that much more difficult when I have to deal with medical insensitivity."

"I understand," Dr. Wicha says compassionately. "I'll make certain the doctor involved knows how she effected you."

"Thank you," I reply gratefully. "That will be helpful."

"I see you are reading "Getting Well Again," Dr. Wicha says with a smile. "What do you think of it?"

"It gives me hope," I answer. "It helps me feel I have some measure of control over this disease. It shows me that the mind-body connection can help heal cancer, and that I can help that healing along."

I look at him to gauge his response. Is it asking too much to want him to agree?

"What do you think?" I ask cautiously.

"I believe there is a strong mind-body connection," Dr. Wicha replies, "and that the mind can have a positive effect on the body, and its ability to heal."

I do not know I have been holding my breath until it comes rushing out noisily. I pick up the two books by Dr. Bernie Siegel lying besides me, and show them to Dr. Wicha.

"Good books," he says, nodding his head. "I've read them. Read them carefully. They contain a lot of good information you can use."

"I will," I promise. "I most definitely will."

To this day, I doubt if Dr. Wicha has any idea how that Friday evening conversation comforted, supported, and strengthened my resolve to heal. It came at a time when I desperately needed the medical profession to treat me with compassion and respect, but most importantly, to offer me the gift of hope. Sometimes, God sends an angel in the guise of a doctor.

CHAPTER 8

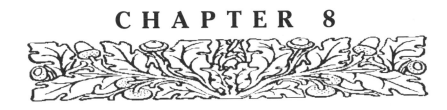

From Hope to Despair

Saturday morning arrives. My room begins filling with family and friends. The phone rings continuously. It is apparent that many calls have been made between yesterday and today, resulting in an outpouring of love that threatens to overwhelm me. As Saturday turns into Sunday, and still people come and go, I realize a group decision has been made. I am to spend the weekend surrounded by unconditional love. Despite what news Monday may bring, I am being given massive infusions of love, to strengthen my ability to handle anything. I feel such love and gratitude toward this outpouring of affection and support, that tears of joy run freely down my face throughout the weekend.

The weekend is also special in a different way. Sunday is Elyssa's twenty fourth birthday, which we celebrate with a birthday cake and a multitude of presents. Stan and I, Sharon and Chuck, Brent, Tracy, Jennifer and her future husband Jon, and Jeff, the man who brings such happiness to Elyssa's life, and whom she will ultimately marry, are in attendance. We noisily sing Happy Birthday to Elyssa, who laughingly makes a wish, and blows out the candles on her cake.

"My wish has to do with you," Elyssa says smilingly. "I can't tell you what it is, but I'm sure you can guess."

"Thank you sweetheart," I answer, deeply moved. "Birthday wishes are very special. Usually they come true."

"I know mine will," Elyssa adamantly replies.

I watch as Jeff moves closer, take Elyssa's hand in his, and gently squeezes it. I am very fond of Jeff, and have noticed on more than one occasion, the laughter and light he adds to Elyssa's life. It will be especially welcome, in the difficult times that lie ahead.

A YEAR OF MIRACLES

As day follows night, so Monday follows Sunday, and the day I have been trying to fortify myself against begins. I am alone in my room, just having finished breakfast, when I learn the results of the latest rib biopsy. The cancer cells are anaplastic, which means they are not well differentiated. However, they have tested negative for multiple myeloma. Given the size of the tumor on the kidney, and the metastasis to the liver and bone, which is not uncommon for kidney cancer, there is unanimous medical agreement as to my diagnosis. I am classified as having advanced metastasized renal cell carcinoma, more commonly called kidney cancer. As I hear those dreaded words pronounced, like a candle in the wind, the tiny flame of hope that burns deep within my heart is extinguished. There is no appeal. The sentence has been handed down. How I respond to it, is up to me.

I would like to be able to say my faith and trust in God is strong, unbending, and unshakable at that traumatic moment, but that would not be the truth. I can recall only one other time in my life, where I feel more abandoned and alone than I do on that April spring morning, facing a probable death sentence. As desperately as I long to turn to God for comfort, protection, and assurance, my fear and terror block the way. I am lost in a maze of my own making, unable to navigate my way to God. To this day, I do not know how long I remain gripped in an agony of terror so dismal, so primitive, so incapacitating, that I am rendered both senseless and immobile.

The ringing of the phone penetrates the thick fog that surrounds me. As fate would have it, it is Dr. Death.

"I hear you are very angry with me," a soft voice says. "I am sorry I upset you so badly."

"You were right," I dully reply.

I am too shattered to feel either anger towards her, or to take pleasure in the apology she offers. All I want is to disappear.

"I'm sorry I am," she answers.

"Me too," I manage to respond.

"I'd still like to be your primary physician," she begins.

I cut her off in mid sentence.

"That won't be possible," I say stiffly. "My answer is still no."

I hang up the phone, and pull the bedcovers over my head. Squeezing my eyes as tightly shut as I can, I float out of my body, and finally disappear.

Sometime later, I become aware that the sound of the television in the next room is blaringly loud. Despite my desire to do otherwise, I am unable to keep the words from penetrating my mind. In a hushed tone, the announcer informs the world that Michael Landon has been diagnosed with advanced pancreatic cancer. His prognosis is grim. I flinch in pain for Michael, and for his family. Unfortunately, I am no stranger to pancreatic cancer. Memories of my own beloved mother flood my mind, bringing tears to my eyes. I recall how valiantly my mother fought to live, yet how tragically she died from this relentless killer, just five short months after her initial diagnosis. Michael's voice comes into my room, strong, determined, and clear. He wants everyone to know he will fight this cancer. He will not give up. He will do everything within his power to live. His courageous words jar me back to reality.

"Me too Michael," I say out loud. "May we both survive."

I do not use the phone to call anyone. I need time alone to absorb the news, to process it my own way. Time to say the words out loud. To taste the bitterness on my tongue. To hear the words escape my mouth, and linger on the air currents. Over and over I chant, kidney cancer, renal cell carcinoma, kidney cancer, renal cell carcinoma, until I no longer cringe from the spoken word. I am somewhat calmer by the time I finish, but it is only a temporary placebo.

My friend Suzanne is visiting, shaken by my diagnosis, but nonetheless trying to be as positive and comforting as she can. I am feeling unusually detached. Almost as if the person we are talking about is someone else. There is a knock on the door, and Dr. Chang enters, introduces himself as a surgical oncologist, and quickly gets down to business.

"I'm here because you have kidney cancer," he begins, "and I think I might be able to help you."

I grab hold of the word help, as I simultaneously recall that this is the doctor Norm talked with me about.

"How can you help me?" I ask, as Suzanne reaches for a pad and a pen, and sits poised to write down the information.

"To begin with, by surgically removing your cancerous left kidney," Dr. Chang responds. "At that time I would also biopsy the growth on your liver."

"How long would that take?" I interject.

"In total, we are looking at a four to five hour surgical procedure, followed by a hospital stay of about a week. Then after a three to four week recuperation at home, you would return to the hospital and begin the experimental adaptive immunotherapy treatments. However, that would only happen if you meet all the protocol requirements."

Protocol requirements. Experimental adaptive immunotherapy. It all sounds like a foreign language to me, but a language that I promise myself I will master.

"What are the protocol requirements?" I ask with trepidation.

"You have to be in good physical health," Dr. Chang answers.

"Except for this cancer, I am very strong and healthy," I reply, "and I know the cancer doesn't disqualify me."

"It just might," Dr. Chang gently states. "It will depend upon some further tests. In order to be admitted to this program, you have to meet four specific requirements. The first is that your remaining right kidney be completely functional and cancer free. The second is that the main blood vessel in your abdomen be cancer free. The third is that the arteries through which the blood flows to your left kidney, be cancer free. The fourth is that the cancer has not metastasized to your brain, because the Interleukin 2 we will be using does not cross over to the brain."

I am floored. I have not even considered that I may have additional tumors. This possibility brings a new wave of terror, that I fight hard to keep under control.

"What happens after I pass your tests with flying colors, and am admitted to your protocol?" I ask, with much more assurance than I am actually feeling.

Dr. Chang hears my fighting spirit, looks closely at me, and smiles.

"It is a multiple step process," he responds. "The first part is the removal and storage of your kidney, which will be used in the making of a cancer fighting vaccine. Then after recuperating from surgery, you will come to the hospital as an outpatient. At that time, you will receive inoculations in the area of both your left and right groin. This area will become very inflamed over the next ten days, but that is a desirable outcome of the inoculation."

"You will return to outpatient surgery, and under a local anesthetic, we will remove the treated lymph nodes from your groin. We will introduce them to the radiated kidney cancer cells, and attempt to grow them. This part is very experimental. Sometimes, we can grow them strong enough and in sufficient quantity, so that we can use them. When we can, we call them "LAK" Cells, or in technical terms Leukocyte Activated Killer cells. They are cells from your own body that have been trained in the laboratory to target and kill your cancer cells. The harvesting of the LAK cells can take three to four weeks, and sometimes even longer. At that point, we will admit you to the hospital, and reinfuse these programmed killer cells into your body. We will follow that up with fifteen infusions of a biological immune enhancing agent called Interleukin 2, every eight hours for the next five days."

"During this treatment you may experience the shakes, low blood pressure, nausea, itching, fluid retention, a weight gain of up to twenty pounds, and possibly other less common though more serious symptoms. These symptoms will begin to disappear upon completion of the treatment. Then a month after we have treated you, we will do another scan to see if the tumors have responded. If you respond favorably, we will continue to treat you every few months."

"Dr. Chang, how do your patients respond?" I ask somewhat nervously.

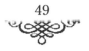

"Some have shown no change, while others have shown some shrinkage of their tumor mass," he replies. "It is about fifty-fifty."

"Have you had any patient whose tumors have completely disappeared?"

I ask the question with trepidation.

"It's a new study," he begins, "and I only have treated a small number of patients, but to answer your question, no I haven't."

My face falls, and Dr. Chang notices it.

"However," he continues, "at the National Institutes of Health, where the study has been going on considerably longer, there have been a very small number of patients for whom all traces of tumor have disappeared."

My heart does a somersault. It has been done before. It can be done again. I can be the one to do it.

"Dr. Chang," I say, smiling the first hopeful smile of this day, "I'll make a deal with you. You help make me cancer free, and I'll help make you famous."

"I'd like that," Dr. Chang responds. "I hope to see that happen."

"It will," I reply. "I'm counting on it."

It only takes a short while for me to read between the lines and to realize the implications to what Dr. Chang has told me. When I do, my euphoria is replaced by a full blown panic attack. I'm going to die, I think. Unless there is a miracle, and I am that one or two in a hundred, I'm dead. As if in slow motion I see my life receding, moving further and further away from those I love. I try with all my might to hold on, but I am wrenched away from all that matters. Sweat pours from my body, leaving damp puddles on the hospital sheets. It is more than I can handle, and I feel something buried deep inside me snap. Suddenly Stan is by my side, wiping my brow, whispering endearments as I, a trapped wild animal, moan and thrash about in bed.

The door opens, and yet another doctor enters.

"I'm Dr. Boxer," I hear a calm voice say, "and I'm here to discuss radiating your left leg."

"I don't want it. Get out," I yell.

"It will speed the healing," the voice replies.

"Everybody wants a piece of me," I scream.

"I want to help you." The voice is soft and warm.

"Nobody can help me. I'm going to die," I shout. "Why don't I just get a gun, and put myself out of my misery now?"

I hear footsteps moving away from my bed and out the door.

I feel Stan's arms encircle me.

"I want to live," I sob. "God, where are You? I want to live."

CHAPTER 9

Keep Your Spirits Up

It strikes me as odd that I awaken Tuesday morning, with the full knowledge that I have a very uncertain life span, yet, relatively speaking, feeling peaceful and centered in trust. My desire to live, and my commitment to do all in my power to overcome this dreaded disease, has only grown stronger during a long and sleepless night.

I am aware of wanting the kind of control over my life which allows me to live to an advanced and healthy old age. Choosing when I am ready to die. Dying a welcomed, and painless death. Yet, it appears the hand I have been dealt is strikingly in opposition to that which I desire. It is true that my attitudes, my beliefs, my fighting spirit, and my ongoing will to live are all positive attributes that help strengthen the life force. So are the prayers, love and support of family and friends, as well as the medical treatments available to me. However, in the deepest recesses of my heart, I know when all is said and done, it will be God who will decide when I return home. And I intuitively sense that my ultimate spiritual challenge is to relinquish control, and strive to develop complete trust and faith in God's Will for me.

My fear, though more suppressed today, lies just barely below the surface, and I find myself tip-toeing around it. This fear is to become a troublesome, ongoing, unwelcome companion, vying for dominance with the faith and trust I so desperately seek to strengthen. Over time, I will learn ways to minimize my fear, and maximize my trust and faith, but for now in order to remain functional, I find that suppression is my best defense.

The door to my room opens, and for the first time I see the face that matches the voice from yesterday. It is a kind, gentle and caring face.

"I thought you might be ready to talk about radiation today," Dr. Boxer begins. Although, I know given the circumstances, my response from yesterday is understandable, I feel acutely embarrassed. Dr. Boxer senses this.

"Don't concern yourself about yesterday," she continues in the kindest of voices, putting me instantly at ease. "I'm glad to see you are doing so much better today."

"I'm hanging in there, but it's touch and go," I admit.

"As it should be," she responds. "The news you were given takes some time to absorb and digest. I'd say you are doing remarkably well."

I like her, I think to myself. I can work with her.

"How can radiation help my leg?" I ask.

"It will help speed the healing process. You will feel less pain, and you will be able to walk without crutches considerably sooner," she replies.

"Is it painful?" I ask.

"Not at all," she answers.

"Can I also have my second and seventh ribs radiated?"

"Why?" she questions gently.

"If I agree to radiation, I would just as soon radiate all the cancerous areas," I explain.

"I would have to make certain Dr. Chang approves," she responds. "In order to be a candidate for immunotherapy, there has to be at least one tumor that can be followed for response to the treatment. I don't see why it can't be the liver tumors, but Dr. Chang is the final authority."

"Will radiation destroy my rib tumors?" I hold my breath, waiting for Dr. Boxer to answer.

"It might, but I don't know how long it will last," she replies looking directly at me. "Radiation is not usually known to be effective with kidney cancer."

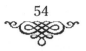

"If Dr. Chang agrees to it, I want do it anyhow," I say quietly. "Miracles do happen."

Dr. Boxer smiles and nods her head in agreement.

"You are right," she gently responds. "Miracles do happen."

Three out of the four tests Dr. Chang orders take place today. In the late morning, I am eased onto a mobile hospital bed, and transported to the basement for a kidney scan. While I lie waiting in line, behind half a dozen patients also waiting to be scanned, a young doctor approaches my bed. He introduces himself as a psychiatrist.

"How are you feeling?" he asks.

"Cold. It's chilly down here. I could use another blanket," I answer.

He tries again.

"I mean about your diagnosis."

"How do you think I'm feeling?" I ask him.

"That's what I'm trying to find out," he replies.

"Shocked. Scared. Like it's a bad dream, and if I try hard enough I'll wake up. And when I do, everything will be like it was before this nightmare began. Except, I can't wake up," I sadly lament.

"Do you have thoughts of hurting yourself?" he asks, gazing intently at me.

"No," I reply indignantly. "I'm hurting enough."

"You were heard saying some things yesterday, that leads me to believe you might try to take your life." He is not asking a question. He is stating a fact.

"Look," I say feeling my anger surface, "I was given a probable death sentence yesterday. I wasn't in my right mind."

"Well," he queries pointedly, "are you?"

I am cold, I am angry, and now I am also exasperated.

"Am I what?" I respond in a raised voice.

"Are you planning on getting a gun and shooting yourself?" he asks, watching me closely for a response.

"No," I yell, "I'm planning on beating this cancer and living. Now, if you really want to help me, get me another blanket. It's freezing down here."

A YEAR OF MIRACLES

In the afternoon, the arteriogram to check my arteries, and the interior vena cava to check my main blood vessel, are performed in quick succession. They are both extremely painful and uncomfortable procedures, and I am delighted to have them behind me. Now the time of waiting for the results of the first three tests begins in earnest.

Before going to bed, I meditate and then ask for a message.

"God," I pray, "what would you have me know?"

I focus on the question, reach into my bag of Runes, and withdraw one. It is the Rune called Jera, the Rune of Harvest, Fertile Season, One Year. The message is as follows:

> "A Rune of beneficial outcomes, Jera applies to any activity or endeavor to which you are committed. Receiving this Rune encourages you to keep your spirits up. Be aware, however, that no quick results can be expected. A span of time always is involved, hence the key words "one year," symbolizing a full cycle of time before the reaping, the harvest, the deliverance."
>
> "You have prepared the ground and planted the seed. Now you must cultivate with care. To those whose labor has a long season, a long coming to term, Jera offers encouragement of success. Know that the outcome is in the keeping of Providence and continue to persevere."
>
> "Remember the farmer who was so eager to assist his crops that he went out at night and tugged on the new shoots. There is no way to push the river, equally you cannot hasten the harvest. Be mindful that patience is essential for the recognition of your own process which, in it's own season, leads to the harvest of the self."

I feel an incredible sense of relief as I absorb the message. A quickening of my faith and trust in God, and a diminishing

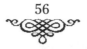

of my fear. I fall asleep easily, and sleep soundly through the night.

Wednesday begins with good news, as I hear from Dr. Chang that all three tests show no signs of cancer. Only one last hurdle remains, one final test to get through, before I am accepted into the program. The head scan is set for Thursday morning, and then after almost two weeks in the hospital, I can finally go home. In the meantime, preparations are taking place for both surgery and radiation. I will be taken down this afternoon for a simulation of the radiation. During the simulation, the precise areas and angles at which I will receive the radiation treatments will be pinpointed. Afterwards, those areas will be marked with small permanent tattoos. I am assured they will blend and look like beauty marks. They will hardly be noticeable. The following week I will begin a series of five megadose radiation treatments, one each morning for five mornings.

Dr. Chang agrees to having my second and seventh ribs treated with radiation. Using CAT scans, he will chart any changes in the size of the liver tumors. This method will allow him to determine the effectiveness of immunotherapy.

"Surgery is scheduled for April 30th," Dr. Chang says.

I quickly calculate. I will have eighteen days at home, before returning to the hospital. Enough time I hope to be fully prepared.

I have one major scare during the day, when I am taken to opthamology to have my eyes examined. There I learn, that a rare, familial, genetic form of kidney cancer can be identified through an eye examination. If I have this kind of kidney cancer, it will mean that my children are also carriers of this gene.

"Not my children," I pray silently. "Please God, spare my children."

After an hour that feels like a long day, my eyes are pronounced healthy and free of this genetic defect.

Gratitude courses through every pore in my body.

"Thank You God," I say fervently. "Thank You for sparing my children."

A YEAR OF MIRACLES

Early Thursday morning, I am taken to radiology for the head scan. This is the last hurdle I have to overcome, before gaining admittance to Dr. Chang's program. It is also a welcome ending, for as soon as this test is completed, I will be discharged from the hospital. Finally, I can return home. Upon discharge, I am handed a sheet of Do's and Don'ts and a home exercise program for the total hip replacement surgery, which I almost have forgotten about, due to the trauma of my cancer diagnosis. In part, it goes as follows:

1- Don't lean too far forward when sitting or standing.
2- Don't turn or roll your leg in.
3- Don't cross your legs. Keep your knees apart.
4- Do stay off your stomach until further advised by your doctor.
5- Do continue to use your crutches.
6- Don't drive a car until advised by your doctor.
7- Do not take a shower until your stitches are out. You may not sit in the tub, until advised by your doctor.
8- Do continue to do the exercises you have been shown, until discontinued by your doctor.

I read the instructions and laugh out loud. After all I have been through, this is like leaving graduate school, and returning to nursery school. I am supposed to follow this advice until two weeks from now, when Dr. Compassion will remove my stitches. Then, he will let me know in his own inimitable way, what I can and cannot do. However, I plan on breaking one of the rules as soon as I possibly can.

CHAPTER 10

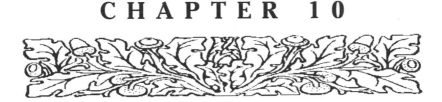

I Shed My Light on Thee

Whoever coined the expression, "Be it ever so humble, there's no place like home," certainly knew what they were talking about. I am ecstatic to return to my home. So many memories are contained within these walls. Fifteen years of love, laughter and tears. This is the home I purchased shortly after Norm and I divorced. Fresh out of graduate school. A single mother of three young children. Beginning a professional career and single parenthood simultaneously. This is the home where I gained emotional and financial independence. Where I learned to be self sufficient, and developed trust in my ability to depend on myself. Where my spiritual nature blossomed and flourished. Where my children grew to adulthood. Where I fell in love again, gave my heart freely, and learned about interdependence. This home mirrors the woman I have finally become.

My joy is even more pronounced by the reception that awaits us as Stan and I enter the house. We are greeted by balloons, flowers, and a banner designed by my friend Larry proclaiming Welcome Home Susan. I am treated to a flurry of happy barks, a wagging tail, and many wet kisses from Mocha. Shanti, only momentarily meows her displeasure at my absence, before settling contentedly on my lap, motor purring overtime. I sit on the couch happily, listening as my home settles around me. There is nowhere I can think of that I would rather be.

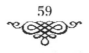

A YEAR OF MIRACLES

It has been decided that Susan will stay with me tonight, and Rose will drive in from Kalamazoo and spend the following night. Rose and I have been fast friends since the summer of 1975, when we meet at Tuwaqachi, a Gestalt community for residents and guests. Both newly separated, both single parents of three young children, a bond born of our mutual struggles, determination, sorrows, triumphs, and joy unites us. Though we live on opposite sides of the state, we have remained involved in one another's lives. From these early beginnings, a solid friendship has formed, which only grows stronger with the passage of time. I am looking forward to seeing Rose, spending quality time with her, and basking in her maternal nurturance. After that I expect to be able to go solo.

My first night home I have a disturbing dream, in which a doctor stands by the side of my bed, and informs me he has bad news to relay. I awaken at 5:00 a.m., drenched in a pool of fear, terrified the results of the brain scan will prove cancerous. Taking some deep breaths, I somehow manage to calm myself. Connecting with God's presence, I am able to fall into an uneasy sleep.

As soon as I awaken, I call Dr. Chang's office for the results of the scan, and am told they will be available later that day. Feeling unsettled, I draw a Rune. In my fear I can interpret it either way, but make myself view it in a positive light.

Still experiencing uneasiness, I call Silent Unity and ask them to pray with me. Silent Unity maintains a twenty four hour prayer vigil, and their prayer room is open day and night. People throughout the world call or write, requesting prayer for all manners of needs, either for themselves or their loved ones. This is just the first of many times I will call Silent Unity. The kind, compassionate woman who speaks with me calms my fears. She helps me remember God's Light, Love, and Power are active in my life. This is a timely reminder, for when I am one with that knowing, no matter what else may be happening, I am centered in peace.

Dr. Chang calls with the confirmation that my brain scan is cancer free, and I am officially accepted into the program. I have such strong and positive feelings about immunotherapy, and believe I will be that one or two in a hundred.

Responding to a knock at the door, I am greeted by Esther Goldstein and three of her children. Esther, the wife of Rabbi Aahron Goldstein, the religious leader of Chabad House is well known for her good deeds or "mitzvahs," as they are called in Judaism. Stan, who is a member of the congregation and very close to the whole family, has spoken with Esther and Aahron about my situation. Besides praying for my recovery, Esther has taken it upon herself to visit, and offer spiritual comfort. Friday evening marks the start of the Sabbath, and Esther brings a challah [a braided bread] she has baked for the Sabbath meal. She also suggests I pray a special Jewish prayer daily, in both Hebrew and English. It is a prayer of giving thanks to God for bestowing goodness upon me. I immediately agree. To this day, I say this prayer upon rising. It has become part of a daily ritual that is as natural to me as breathing.

Friday evening, for the first time in too many years, I reverently place the Sabbath candles into my grandmother's silver candle sticks. Saying the blessing for the Sabbath, I light the candles, and pray for a healing. A sense of hope and well being envelops me, and I marvel at how strong a connection I feel to my Jewish roots. The Light from the Sabbath candles ignites the Light in my Soul.

Saturday morning, Stan drives me to my first acupuncture session with Charles Lincoln, a close family friend. Stan and I have talked about acupuncture numerous times these past few weeks. I know from Stan's own personal experience with acupuncture, he thinks very highly of Charles' abilities. I am somewhat nervous, for I do not relish having needles stuck into my skin. Still, I am more than willing to try whatever may prove helpful. Charles initial assessment is two fold. He will use acupuncture to reduce the pain from the hip surgery, and to strengthen my body in readiness for the kidney surgery to follow. Following kidney surgery, he will continue using acupuncture to reduce pain, promote healing, strengthen my remaining kidney, and build up my weakened immune system. I am pleasantly surprised at finding acupuncture is not painful, and actually induces a state of relaxation. I leave with the first of many bottles of Chinese herbs, a good feeling about Charles and this treatment, and an appointment for the following week.

That evening, Stan and I go out to dinner and celebrate my homecoming. I find myself feeling human once again. Mingling with other people. Being a part of everyday life. No one pays undue attention to my use of crutches. I am just one of the crowd. No more or no less. I am learning that one of the hardest things about having cancer is guarding against becoming so caught up in my illness, that I lose track of an outside world. Back home, Stan teaches me how to work with my cells on a cellular level through a specific visualization. In using this visualization, my healthy cells remain healthy, and my diseased cells are destroyed. It is a technique Stan discovered fifteen years ago, while learning to control his hay fever. I don't know if I can do it Stan's way, or if I need to make modifications of my own, but I willingly give it a try.

Relaxed, and delighted at being together, we find ourselves cuddling, and sharing some much needed intimacy. It gives me pleasure to give Stan pleasure. I am taped and too physically limited to have it fully reciprocated. However, the touching, hugging, and kissing brings out the woman in me. Aware that it has been too long since she has shown up, I joyously welcome her back.

That night I have two dreams. In the first one, which plays continually throughout the night, I am outside my body fixing its faulty wiring, by redirecting the cancer killing cells. As new bodily connections are established, the cancer killing cells rapidly multiply, attacking and destroying the cancer cells. As this mind-body connection continues, my immune system grows stronger. The stronger it becomes, the more cancer killing cells it produces. These cancer killing cells significantly outnumber and completely destroy all the cancer cells in my body, and I am cancer free.

In the second dream, I am sitting in bed, reading a book, and laughing. As I play with the words, rearranging them in different sequences, I feel happy and content. I look toward my right, and sitting at my bedside is a stern, grim faced doctor. He stares at me as if I have lost my mind.

"Don't you realize the seriousness of your situation?" his somber presence implies.

I look away from him and towards the door. I smile as Susan and Marilyn walk in. They immediately begin playing with the words, rearranging the sequence, and changing its meaning. All three of us are laughing, acting silly and childlike.

"Go down and be with the children," they urge. "That's where you belong."

"I can't," I answer, pointing to the stern faced doctor. "He thinks I am sick and belong here. But I know I would be much better off if I were with the children."

I interpret this dream as a clear message that however long my life span, I need to live it with childlike wonder, laughing, loving, playing, creating new meaning, and enjoying the time I have, rather than living a grim and somber life, waiting to die and afraid to live. I am flesh and blood. I love. I feel. I think. I am who I was before this diagnosis. Active. Alert. Alive. I vow to continue to live that way for all the remaining days of my life.

After an early morning visit from my friend Joan, who has generously volunteered to food shop for as long as I need her to, I have an insight about how life threatening illness has a way of creating everyday miracles. I am connecting more deeply and genuinely with people than ever before. These connections are so powerful as to leave no doubt as to their authenticity. It appears that people around me, aware of their own mortality, are letting their own light shine through. In doing so, they are becoming more of who they really are. During these past few days, as I sit with family and friends, and we open our hearts to one another, I can sense the whole room aglow with God's Love and Light.

A YEAR OF MIRACLES

Dr. Boxer's call at 10:30 p.m. awakens me from a sound sleep. My initial reaction is one of fear, for I have become conditioned to hearing bad news from doctors. This is different. Dr. Boxer, has just gotten the x-rays of my ribs, and has started reviewing them. She is concerned about how close the tumor on my seventh rib is to my spinal cord. She wonders if it is pressing on my spinal cord, causing me difficulty with urination or bowel movements. She is also considering using a more aggressive approach in radiating this area. For once I am not alarmed. I have known for some time of the tumor's proximity to my spine. I assure Dr. Boxer that if anything, I urinate too frequently, and since discontinuing the use of codeine for pain, my bowels work fine. As for using a more aggressive approach to combat the tumor, I am all for that.

Reflecting on our conversation, I recognize that there are an abundance of miracles occurring in my life that I have overlooked. Neither the rib tumors nor the kidney tumor are affecting nearby organs, and despite the cancer, my body works fine. I see how blind I have been in not recognizing the little miracles that are part of each day. If only my eyes were fully open, how many miracles would I see? Often it is the big, knock your socks off miracles that I so focus on, that I don't notice, appreciate, or give thanks for the smaller, less spectacular miracles God blesses my life with. By gaining an awareness of these miracles, and opening myself to God's loving plan, I can strengthen my faith, diminish my fears, and step by step, in partnership with God, create the miracle I so longingly desire. I make a decision to consciously take note of all the miracles occurring in my life, and thank God for each and every one of them.

It is very early in the morning, a time I usually sleep through. However, today I am wide awake waiting for Tracy's arrival, for she is to bring me to my 7:00 a.m. radiation appointment. Tracy usually sleeps through the early morning as well, by arranging college classes for later in the day. I am pleased Tracy and Sharon will be alternating mornings this week, and that she won't be rising this early every day. I feel prepared, and only the slightest bit nervous. I have been using a visualization tape to help prepare for the radiation treatments. I am visualizing my friends the golden rays entering my body, and causing the cancer cells to explode, while leaving my other cells unharmed.

As I enter the waiting room, I am amazed at the number of people in need of treatment. All ages. All stages. From infant, to young adult, to senior citizen, they are all represented. Women. Men. Children. All part of a group, none of us would willingly choose to belong to. All hoping that this treatment will help. That it will destroy the cancer. That a miracle will occur. My name is called, and Tracy and I follow the nurse through the swinging doors, down the hallway, and into the women's dressing room. I change into a hospital gown, kiss Tracy goodbye, walk down another hallway, my crutches moving double-time, and enter the radiation room. The heavy steel doors shut behind me.

The actual treatment goes amazingly fast. I am positioned on the table by a radiation technician, so that my cancerous ribs and hip are aligned with the machine. I look up at the massive machine. It looks down at me.

"Hello Goldie," I whisper. Not the most original name, but it personalizes the piece of metal above me.

The technician makes some last minute adjustments, and leaves the room. The door closes with a heavy thud. I am completely alone. Suddenly, I hear the disembodied voice of the technician through a speaker.

"I'll let you know when to lay absolutely still," she announces, "and when you can move again. It is very important to follow my instructions exactly. It won't take long. I can hear you, so please let me know that you can hear me."

"I hear you," I answer.

"Good," she says. "We are about to begin. Lie still, and don't move."

I hear a dull whirring sound coming from the machine. I visualize golden rays entering my body, targeting the cancer cells. I see the cancer cells explode and land in a pile on the floor. Suddenly, quite unbidden and totally unrehearsed, a broom and dustpan come dancing into the room. Not your ordinary broom and dustpan either. Both resemble cartoon characters, and have arms, legs, and large smiling faces. The broom sweeps the cancer cells into the dustpan. The dustpan pushes a button on its handle, and a large, clear plastic top descends, trapping and covering the exploded cancer cells. Mission completed, the broom and dustpan, dance out of sight. I hear giggling and see a little girl, dark ringlets framing her chubby face, jumping up and down, her body wiggling with delight. She is about four years old, and I recognize myself, from a picture taken of me at that age. I make a mental note to remove that picture from my photograph album, and place it where I see it every day.

The door opens, and I return to the room with a start.

"You can go now," the technician says, helping me off the table. "We'll see you same time tomorrow."

I return to the dressing room, change into my clothes, and find Tracy in the waiting room.

"I'm starving. Let's go to Angelo's for breakfast," I say. "I have a craving for raisin French toast."

I will find that this imaging sequence with my little girl will grow stronger with each additional radiation treatment. I will find that instead of feeling tired from the radiation, as I have been warned I might, I will become more and more energized. I will find myself ravenous after each treatment, and five mornings in a row, I will devour Angelo's raisin French toast with gusto. I will also find myself at the end of the treatment hugging Dr. Boxer and promising to return for a visit at the end of five years, healthy, healed, and very much alive. And I will find Dr. Boxer returning my hug, and telling me she expects to see me.

Nancy, Betty, Karen, and I are holding our first Creating Results business meeting at my home since the start of my illness. I have warm feelings towards all three, but share a special bond with Betty, a member of Gwen's group whom I have become very close to, and who is a tremendous support in my fight to regain my health. We are taking a short break, and drinking tea when another miracle occurs. Karen, a registered nurse, suggests that I contact Dr. James Thomas, at The Center For Contemporary Medicine, a multidisciplinary practice for optimal health, located all of three miles from my home. She has worked with him, and feels I would appreciate his approach to the treatment of cancer, which is biopsychosocial, more commonly referred to as the mind-body connection. This approach focuses on the interactions between the psychological self, the biological body, and the individual's social and cultural environments. In addition to being Director of the Center, Dr. Thomas has been an Associate Professor of Pharmacology at Wayne State University, a Research Associate at the National Institutes of Health, and has over ten years experience facilitating groups for women with breast cancer, with impressive results. I am convinced without seeing Dr. Thomas, that I want him on my team. I call his office, and manage to arrange an appointment for the following afternoon.

Dr. Thomas, or James as I take to calling him, wins me over immediately.

"You are an individual, not a statistic," James stresses as I sit in his office. "So do yourself a big favor, and ignore the statistics. You are unique. There is no one quite like you, so the way you respond will be unlike anyone else with the same disease. You are an active participant in your own recovery. You are not a victim, and don't let anyone tell you otherwise."

"We are going to get on famously," I think to myself.

" I believe completely in your innate ability to effect your recovery. I see my role as assisting you in that process through our entering into a mutual partnership. So why don't we begin to discover how we can best work together, to help enhance your natural ability to heal." James finishes speaking, and smiles at me.

"I'm ready," I say, and smile back.

I like James' philosophy. I like his easy, relaxed, sensitive manner. And I am very impressed by just how knowledgeable he is. About medicine. About psychology. About meditation. About visualization, and guided imagery. About prayer. About spirituality. About exercise. About yoga. About nutrition.

About vitamins. About all the latest research, both traditional, and alternative, in the field of cancer.

"There are three things I would like you to start doing right away," James says. "The first is a specific visualization called, "Awakening Your Inner Physician." I would like you to record it in your own voice, and play it every morning. The visualization will help you connect more deeply to your source of inner intuitive knowing, which is essential to the process of personal empowerment and healing."

I nod. I am in complete agreement, and already deeply connected to the Source from which all else flows.

"The second, involves some deep breathing and stretching exercises, that will help your body stay healthy, well oxygenated, and supple. You can stretch, even with the hip replacement," he adds. "We'll just modify the exercise."

"Okay," I say. "No problem."

"An added benefit is that cancer cells can't live in an oxygen rich environment."

"Sounds good to me," I respond.

"The third combines breath work, the inhalation and exhalation, in combination with a 'think-see, think-speak' sequence. I will teach you how to do that. It will probably feel uncomfortable at first, but will become natural rather quickly. I would like you to work with this technique, and see if you can begin to shut off the blood supply to the tumors in your kidney and liver. If tumors are totally deprived of blood, they will shrivel and die," James explains. "Do this three or four times a day, ten minutes each time."

"I'll try," I say. "I'll do my best."

"I know you will," James responds. "I can tell that about you, already."

As I walk into the house, I hear the phone ring. It is Gwen calling from California, with a message she has channeled, and wishes to share. Gwen has been told that I have great powers to reverse mutations, and an increased natural ability to do so. Over this past year, a strong foundation upon which I can now build has emerged. It is time to take the next step. Time to prepare, strengthen and nourish myself. Ultimately, there will be a transformation to another dimension for me, but without involving a death. In this dimension, I will have the energy of joy and light continually in my vibrational field. Emerald green is a strong healing color for me, and Gwen urges that I wear it and surround myself with it as frequently as possible. I am to focus on the emerald green vibration every morning at 9:00 a.m., while Gwen will be focusing on it 6:00 a.m. California time. Together, we will work to raise this healing vibration in my energy field.

"Try not to worry," Gwen concludes. "You will heal."

It never ceases to amaze me, how quickly I can shift from hope, faith and trust, to doubt, terror and despair. I can observe the change occurring, yet feel powerless in the moment to alter it. Oftentimes, there is no precipitating factor that creates the change in outlook and attitude. It occurs spontaneously, fueled by an energy beyond my control, and as I get ready for bed, it strikes swiftly and with a powerful fury. I lie awake much of the night, trying to calm my raging emotions, and failing miserably. Exhausted by the struggle, I pray one final time for help in overcoming my inner enemies of doubt, terror, and despair, and at last fall into an uneasy sleep. Only hours later, I awaken with a start, with a message indelibly imprinted upon my mind. On April 20, 1991, at 6:25 a.m., I write the following on the back of the picture taken of me at age four, that is now sitting on my night stand:

> *I shed My Light on thee.*
> *I illuminate thy heart and mind.*
> *Thy body will heal.*
> *Trust in Me.*

As I sit in bed, incredulously reading and rereading the message, I feel a strong and loving connection with God. I know no matter what I go through, no matter how strong my fears and doubts may be, that God's love is constant, and that I will ultimately heal. I want to hold on to this moment forever, to imprint it upon my soul, and feel the joy and gratitude of this knowing. I pray to God, as the source of all good, to help me always remember what I now so clearly know.

A YEAR OF MIRACLES

CHAPTER 11

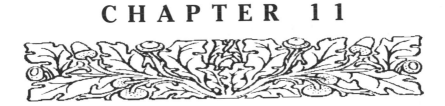

Then Will I Perform Miracles

I frequently find myself thinking of my brother Kal these past few weeks. Five years younger than me, we grow up as children of a devoted, protective, loving mother, whose societal sin is in having divorced a man whose failure as both husband and father is the talk of our close knit family. Kal and I are the only children in our neighborhood, in our school, and it appears to us, in all of Brooklyn, New York, branded by the stigma of divorce. Being different creates a special closeness, and strengthens the bond between us throughout our childhood years. As we grow to adulthood, marry, have children of our own, and physically move a great distance apart, our ongoing contact is limited to occasional cards, calls, and visits. Although, I am less than happy about this situation, I have become complacent, and grown to accept it. Now, with the diagnosis of cancer, I find myself longing for that old closeness and deep connection with my brother Kal.

With some trepidation, I pick up the phone and place a call to Canada. The phone is answered by my sister in law Karen.

"Hi Karen. It's Susan," I quietly say. "I'd like to talk with Kal, if he's around."

Karen can tell something is wrong by the tone of my voice.

"What is it? What's happening?" she asks.

"Karen, please have Kal get on another line. I'll talk with both of you then," I reply.

I hear some talking in the background, and my brother comes on the line.

"Sue, what is going on?" he asks sounding nervous, and calling me by my childhood name.

"Kal, I have advanced kidney cancer," I manage to stammer.

There is the inhalation of breath, and dead silence.

"Kal, did you hear what I said?"

"I'm hoping I heard wrong, but I think I heard right," he answers. "This comes as such a shock, that I'm speechless, and you know I'm never at a loss for words."

"I'm sorry to drop this bombshell on you," I say unhappily.

"Listen Sue," Kal continues, "you are my sister, and I want to be there for you in any way I can. Just tell me how."

"Me too," Karen murmurs.

"You are doing it now, both of you, just by your response." I begin to cry.

"Sue, just listen to me." Kal's voice is strong and clear. "You are going to beat this cancer. I know you. You are a fighter. You are stubborn. You are strong and determined. You were like that as a child, and you are more so now. Sue, you are a winner. You are going to win. The cancer doesn't stand a chance."

"Kal, you don't even know anything about this kind of cancer. How can you be so sure?" I ask.

"I'm going to learn a lot about it," he replies. "You can count on that. What I do know a lot about though is you. And I know that you are going to win this battle. There is no doubt in my mind. No matter what I learn."

"Nor mine," Karen adds. "Kal is right. You are going to overcome this cancer."

"I believe that also," I respond. "At least most of the time."

"Good," they simultaneously reply.

"Now, that that's out of the way, bring us up to date as to what's gone on, and as to what's going to be happening from here on," Kal orders.

"Bossy," I say smiling through my tears, as I begin to fill them in.

Early afternoon, I break the one rule on the list of do's and don'ts, that I have promised to break. After more than three weeks without one, I finally get to do what I have done every day prior to my hospital stay. With Sharon's help, we manage to wrap my left hip and leg in yards of saran wrap, layer it with industrial strength plastic lawn bags, and then seal it with duct tape, so that not a single drop of water can find its way in. I am a strange and sorry looking sight to behold, and we both double over with laughter. At last, the moment I have been waiting for arrives. With assistance from Sharon, I climb into the tub, turn on the shower, and feel the delicious spray of hot water caressing my skin. As I wash the thick patina of the hospital stay off my body, I feel really clean for the first time in weeks. No amount of sponge bathing can do that. My skin glows, and smells fresh, which intensifies my feelings of being healthy. Tonight, when Stan and I come together in love, I can be all woman, and experience the spiritual, emotional, and physical bond that my body, my soul, and I, all hunger for.

Late afternoon, my friend Anne arrives to install the Multi-Pure water system I have purchased. I am excited that I will be drinking filtered water. It seems appropriate that this is happening now, since the kidney also acts as a filter, filtering out waste products. Now the waste products and dangerous chemicals will be removed, both in the water I drink, and through the surgery on my diseased left kidney. I experience this as another affirmation on the road to healing.

Being with Stan tonight leaves me wrapped in a soft, warm, blanket of love.

Stan holds me in a tight embrace, looks into my eyes, then gently moves my head to his chest as he whispers in my ear,

"I very much want you to live for a very long time. I have a vested self interest in that happening."

I look up at him and smile.

"I'll remember that, and hold you to it," I say playfully.

"You'd better," he replies.

We both laugh, and lying side by side, drift into an easy sleep.

A YEAR OF MIRACLES

I dream that night that I have cancer, but despite no guarantee of healing, I am filled with joy. It is one of those dreams that continues throughout the night, with the word joy repeated over and over in my mind while I sleep. I awaken filled with boundless joy and gratitude for the gift of daily life. I begin writing this dream in my journal, but as other sentences appear, fully formed in my minds eye, I write the following instead:

You will know many springtimes
to walk this land
with the one you love.
Hand in hand,
amongst the flowers.
For you are My beloved child,
a fragrant flower,
whose essence will fill
the earth plane
for many long years
to come.

All that I ask you to be,
you already are.
And by becoming yourself
your soul is freed
to do My work.

When belief is born
from the depths of thy heart,
and the words on thy lips
are pure,
then will I come to thee
and perform miracles.

I put down the pen, and look at what I have written. I recognize it as automatic writing. I write frequently, and am quite familiar with the writing process. This is a distinctively different experience. I have not thought of these words. The words have arrived as fully formed sentences. They have come through me, rather than from me. With an abiding sense of gratitude, I joyously give thanks to the One.

Brent stops by in the afternoon to see how I am feeling.

"I'm feeling amazingly good," I say. "I love it when you stop by or call. It makes me happy."

"Well that's easy," he answers.

"What's easy?" I ask.

"Making you happy." He grins the family grin. The one I can never get my fill of seeing on him.

"I'm just a sucker for a good looking guy," I admit.

"Awe Mom," he says rolling his eyes, his grin growing even brighter.

One of my most looked forward to times of the day is in reading the cards and letters of support, encouragement and love that arrive with the mail. Until this verbal outpouring, I do not fully grasp how many people my life is intermingled with, and I am stunned by the sheer magnitude. People I have not thought of telling know, and I realize how immense a network I am a part of. Mail continues to arrive daily from the United States, Canada and Europe. It cheers me, reinforces my efforts to heal, shows me how much I am part of a greater whole, and how very well loved I am.

Adie writes from Boston:

> Dear Mom #2,
> Elyssa has filled me in as to what has been going on. Needless to say I am very sad, for you are a very important person in my life. I know you are a very strong woman in many ways, and that you have lots of supportive, caring people around you. If anyone can beat this, overcome this, you can. I just wanted to let you know my thoughts and energy are with you. I love you very much.

Sheila and I have been dear friends since birth. Our mothers have been close friends since early childhood. More than twenty years ago, Sheila's husband George was diagnosed with Metastatic Melanoma, a frequently fatal form of skin cancer. He has fully recovered, and remains cancer free. Sheila writes from New Jersey:

> "Call anytime you feel like talking, day or night. I'll call you back to keep the phone bill down. And please, when I call, if you don't feel like talking, don't hesitate to say so. I'll understand. My thoughts are with you constantly, along with my love and prayers. All will be well."

Michael, Sheila's twenty one year old son, writes from Spain:

> "I spoke with mom, and she told me of the recent developments in your life. Someone here on another continent is really pulling for you. Just know that. It's easy to see why my mom chose you as one of her best friends, and why you have been so good to me. Keep fighting. I love you."

Kal and Karen, and my nephews Kris and Kirk, write from Canada:

> "Though we may not totally understand everything you're going through, don't ever forget that we'll support you and stand by you always... with all the love a family can give. You will beat this."

Sharon writes:

> "I don't want to think about what life would be like if I didn't share it with you. I just want to make every moment together count. Today and always. I love you so much."

THEN WILL I PERFORM MIRACLES

Rebecca writes from Ann Arbor:

"I'm enclosing a prayer from the Healing Circle ceremony at the Chapel of Love for Spiritual Truth. I really like this part of the Sunday Service. Everyone holds a crystal at the same time they hold hands in a circle. Then they go around and place names of their friends and loved ones into the circle. I've been placing your name in the circle, and will continue to do so. I will be saying this prayer for you daily, and especially on the 30th of April."

PRAYER FOR SPIRITUAL HEALING

I ask the Great Unseen Healing Force
To remove all obstructions
From my mind and body,
And to restore me to perfect health.
I ask this in all sincerity and honesty
And I will do my part.

I ask this Great Unseen Healing Force
To help both present and absent ones
Who are in need of help
And to restore them to perfect health.
I put my trust
In the love and power of God.

Barbara, a friend from Gwen's group, and witness to my pledge to study the element of fire for 3 years, 3 months, 3 weeks, and 3 days writes from San Diego:

"Perhaps, now is the time to turn within to the Eastern Goddesses, Asherah and Sarasvati, you have pledged to honor, and to seek their counsel. They know about pleasure and passion, and how to enjoy and receive life. They are best reached through the physical body. They know about treating the body with gentleness and softness. They know about the voluptuous pleasure in eating an apple and licking the nectar from fingers and lips. They know how important it is for a woman to love her own body with a sweet, accepting love, a deep caring love. Deepen your loving relationship with your own body. Celebrate life. Listen to your body, and it will guide you towards health and wholeness."

Gail, another member of Gwen's group, and a fine musician, writes from Royal Oak, Michigan:

"I've been sending you light and love every day in my meditation, and have dedicated all the music I have been playing to your healing."

Susan writes from Ann Arbor:

"I'm not the only one who loves you so dearly. Besides your family, friends, and Universal Fan Club, so does God. Remember. God's Strength Is Your Strength. Always."

Today's mail also brings information from the American Cancer Society, and the National Cancer Institute on kidney cancer. I am proud of viewing the information in a positive light, instead of panicking as I read the glum statistics, for it would be easy to perceive what I read in a negative light. I remember James' emphatic message, that I am unique and not a statistic, and it helps ease my way. Actually I learn some interesting facts. Only 2% of all cancers are kidney cancer, and it is most common in men. Even more interesting to me is that only 0.7% of all women who are diagnosed with cancer, develop kidney cancer. It seems I am in a very exclusive club. I think about the significance of being part of such a minority, and realize if I were going to play the game of statistics, I would have to conclude that my chances of recovery are significantly greater than my chances ever were of contracting this disease. Arriving at this conclusion fills my soul with laughter, and my heart with renewed hope.

Before going to sleep, I meditate on the meaning of developing such a rare form of cancer, and ask for clarity, but only if it is in my best interest to know. During the night, I receive this message.

"You needed something that would totally claim your attention, in order for you to focus totally on yourself. You get worried, anxious and frightened at times, but don't be. Know you will heal."

I ponder this response. It is true I have a tendency to focus more on the needs of others than on my own needs, as is common for many women. It is also true that since developing cancer, my focus has been almost totally on my healing. Yet, the sense I get regarding this advanced and relatively rare form of cancer, is somehow connected with the medical community. I suspect that my remarkable recovery will generate an inordinate amount of attention and interest in the field of medicine. And ultimately, this will prove beneficial for many others.

What a high I feel today. I am stapleless and weaned from my cane. Dr. Compassion has just informed me in his own inimitable way, that I can walk from here to California and back. Won't Marilyn, June and Gwen be surprised to see me!! I still have some minor limitations. No tying shoes for two more months. No crossing my left leg over my right one. No lying on my right side, because that will leave my left leg unsupported, but other than that almost anything goes. It is the first time in three months that I can walk without crutches or a cane, and I am ecstatic. I do walk with a slight limp, but I am assured that too will disappear. And finally, I can drive my new, beautiful, red Toyota Celica, and reclaim the independence of mobility.

CHAPTER 12

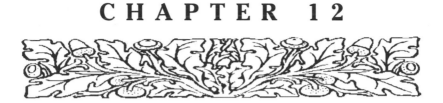

I Love You, I Love You, I Love You

The three weeks spent at home ends all too quickly, and my imminent return to the hospital becomes a current reality. However, this time I am prepared, and know what to do to insure my week long stay will be as healing as possible. On Tuesday, April 30, 1991, Stan, Sharon, and I arrive at the admissions office at the unlikely hour of 6:00 a.m.. Lucky Tuesday is what I call it. Accompanying us is a cart filled with my belongings. Packed to overflowing, it holds my hand stitched butterfly quilt, two butterfly sheets and pillowcases, two plump down pillows, many healing crystals, two large pastel pictures to brighten the drab hospital walls, a tape recorder and tapes, my journal, five bright and cheery nightgowns, assorted photographs of family and friends, and a variety of personal articles for grooming. Nestling inside the oversized purse that sits on top of the cart, are dozens of the cards and letters that mean so much to me, an escape novel, and two inspirational books about people who have healed from terminal cancer.

We sit in the crowded waiting room until my name is called. Following the nurse into a tiny cubicle where I will remain until taken to surgery, I change into a hospital gown and place a cap on my head, tucking my long curly hair inside. My vital signs are monitored, and additional blood is drawn.

"This is the latest in surgical wear," I say with a straight face. "What do you think?"

"It's you," Sharon answers.

"Absolutely," Stan concurs.

We fall suddenly silent. What is there to say that we haven't said at least a hundred times before?

"It's time to go," the nurse says, entering the cubicle unannounced.

I kiss Stan and Sharon, holding them in a tight embrace. It is hard to pull myself away, and copious tears flow down my cheeks.

"It's all right mom. The surgery will go well," Sharon says lovingly. "I'll be waiting in your room. You'll see me as soon as you open your eyes."

"Your room will be so welcoming, that it will remind you of home," Stan assures me. "And of course, I'll be waiting there for you. Remember Susan, God is with you. You are in good hands."

I kiss both of them one last time, as I am wheeled away to surgery.

The ceiling of the operating room is crisscrossed with bright overhead lights, and the brightness hurts my eyes when I glance up. Craning my neck from side to side, I notice that many gowned doctors and nurses are congregated in the center of the room.

"Where is Dr. Chang?" I ask. "I need to talk with him."

A gowned figure separating itself from the group, slowly and steadily moves towards me.

"Hello Susan," Dr. Chang gently says.

"Hello Dr. Chang," I somewhat nervously reply. "I have a special request to make of you. While I am under anesthesia, I would appreciate if you told me the surgery is going well, and that I will heal easily and without complications. I believe that my unconscious mind will receive and respond favorably to a positive message. Will you do that for me?"

"I will." Dr. Chang nods his head in agreement.

"I have another request to make of you," I continue, feeling more at ease given Dr. Chang's previous response. "During surgery, I would prefer any talk around me to be kept positive. I believe that my unconscious mind can be influenced by negative talk, and that can influence my body's ability to recover. I don't know if that is your belief, but I would be grateful if you would honor mine."

"Consider it done," Dr. Chang replies. "Is there anything else?"

"That's all I can think of for now," I answer. "And thank you, Dr. Chang."

"You're welcome Susan." His voice sounds warm and reassuring.

"God," I pray as the anesthesiologist appears at my side, "Into Thy Hands I Commend My Soul. May Thy Will Be Done."

I awaken to a circle of familiar, beloved faces. Stan. Sharon. Elyssa. Brent. Chuck. Jeff. Tracy. Jennifer. Susan. For a moment, I don't know where I am, but then it all comes flooding back.

"The surgery?" I croak. There are tubes running from my nose into my throat, and it hurts to swallow.

"You came through with flying colors Mom," Elyssa answers quickly. "Dr. Chang said the surgery went very well."

"My kidney?"

"Gone into deep freeze, until you have immunotherapy," Brent smilingly replies.

I feel my abdomen through the many layers of bandages and tape. It is extremely tender and sore to the touch.

"I hurt," I say, my voice sounding hoarse.

Someone pushes the button by my bed and a nurse rushes in.

"I'm going to give you a shot for the pain," she explains. "You will feel better in no time."

The needle enters my arm. I sleep.

It is the middle of the night when I awaken, and I can see a sky full of stars from my bed. I lie quietly, letting my eyes adjust to the darkness. I listen to the steady beating of my heart. It soothes and comforts me. Raising my right hand, I see it has an IV in it. I lower it, and trace the embroidered butterflies on my quilt with my fingertips. Slowly, peacefully, I drift into a gentle sleep.

Morning brings with it all the hustle and bustle a busy teaching hospital attracts. I am awakened by morning rounds.

A YEAR OF MIRACLES

"How are you feeling Susan?" Dr. Chang solicitously inquires.

"Very sore. Intermittent pain. Overall not too bad," I respond.

I point to the tubes in my nose and throat.

"What are these for?" I ask.

"For nourishment. After this kind of surgery, you are unable to eat for a few days," Dr. Chang answers. "I know they feel uncomfortable, but they are necessary for your recovery."

"Tell me about the surgery," I say, accepting the need for the tubes.

"It went very well, and was quite uneventful. I removed your diseased kidney, and a portion of one of the tumors on your liver. I sent the liver tumor to the laboratory for a biopsy. It looks like kidney cancer, that has spread to your liver. However, the laboratory report will give us a final diagnosis. We should know within a couple of days," he adds.

We talk a few more minutes, and Dr. Chang leaves the room.

"I guess all that imaging of shutting off the blood supply to my liver hasn't made a difference," I glumly think.

Sunlight streams through the window, and as I look around the room, it illuminates one of the framed pictures on the otherwise sterile hospital wall. It is a large pastel that Stan has drawn from the photograph taken of me at age four. Underneath the picture, in bold letters is printed, "I shed My Light on Thee." The other picture also drawn by Stan, is an even larger framed pastel of my spirit animal, the wolf. I have named him Wolfgang, and he is my guardian and protector. Stan has signed both pictures, using his Hebrew name Simcha, which means Joy. I find this very fitting, since Stan brings so much joy into my life. Stan signs all of his artwork this way. Crystals lying on my night stand catch the morning sun and sparkle gaily. Cards and photographs line the windowsill, and are tacked onto the bulletin board. My butterfly quilt covers me, as my head rests on a butterfly pillowcase. My tape recorder and tapes are within easy reach, and my journal and books are tucked into the night stand. Feelings of safety and security encircle me, as I look about my home away from home.

I am half sitting up in bed, listening to a tape, when Stan enters the room. I am all too aware of my appearance, and feel self conscious about it . My long, curly hair, caked with sweat, is in desperate need of a washing. The tubes running from my nose to throat do little to enhance my overall feelings of femininity. Referring to the dark brown liquid running through them, they will be officially christened "eh-eh tubes" by Pat, later in the day.

Stan appears preoccupied and troubled.

"I can't figure out what's happening," he begins. "I'm just feeling down, depressed, and out of sync."

I look at him amazed. Can he really be that out of touch?

"I think I know what's going on, but I'm not sure you want to know," I respond.

Stan looks into my eyes and swallows hard. "Tell me what you think," he says hesitantly.

I close my eyes. "God help me say this without frightening him," I silently pray.

"Okay," I begin nervously. "I think you are in love with me, and are keeping that knowledge from yourself . I also think you are feeling down and depressed because I have cancer, and you are afraid of losing me."

Stan just stares at me.

"You really think that?" he finally manages to ask.

"I really do," I reply, my voice sounding outwardly strong, though inwardly I am shaking.

"I need some time to think about what you said," Stan responds haltingly. We can talk more about it later." Soon after, he leaves.

"Oh God," I moan. "What did I just do?"

My room is crowded all day, with a steady stream of visitors. Family and friends offer words of encouragement, love, support, and humor. Each time the door opens, my heart races wildly, then resumes its normal rhythm, when I realize it is not Stan. As day turns to night, I resign myself to the fact that Stan will not be returning today. The door opens at 10:00 p.m.. Convinced it is a nurse, I don't even bother turning around.

"I love you," Stan says, striding towards my bed. "I love you, I love you, I love you."

I promptly burst into tears.

Stan reaches for me through the tubes and IV. Somehow we manage to embrace, for it is true that where there's a will, there's a way. When we finally disentangle ourselves, we begin to talk in earnest.

"I thought about what you said all day," Stan begins, "and the longer I thought about it, the more I knew you spoke the truth. I waited until now because I wanted us to be alone when I told you."

"No witnesses," I say.

"Just you, and me, and God," Stan replies.

"Stan, you are not going to lose me. I have even more reason to live now than before." I speak these words as if they are indeed a fact.

Stan covers my hand with both of his. Uninhibited tears flow down his cheeks.

"I never, ever, want to lose you. I want to be with you, forever and a day," he lovingly says.

"We will be." I speak quietly, and with deep conviction. "Our being together is a part of God's plan for us."

"I also believe that." Stan cups my head gently, and looks deeply into my eyes.

"Forever and a day," he says smiling.

I smile back at this beautiful, tender, sensitive, gentle man that I have waited my whole life to love and be loved by.

"Forever and a day," I promise.

Dr. Chang looks puzzled, when he enters my room.

"We have the results of the liver biopsy," he begins, "and it doesn't show cancer. It shows only dead cells, and is the kind of cellular structure I would expect to see in cirrhosis of the liver."

"Dr. Chang, I don't drink," I say. "Never have."

"I don't know what to make of this," Dr. Chang continues. "I am having additional laboratory tests run. If the results remain the same, I will want you to have a liver biopsy. It can be performed on an outpatient basis, and you could leave several hours later. This is highly unusual. I saw that lesion, and it looked exactly like kidney cancer that had spread to the liver."

If my liver is cancer free, then there will be no tumor for Dr. Chang to track, and immunotherapy would no longer be an option, I think .

"Dr. Chang," I ask, "would I be better off having a liver that is cancer free and no immunotherapy, or cancer in the liver and immunotherapy?"

Dr. Chang answers without hesitation. "No cancer in the liver. We can always do immunotherapy, if the need arises."

I like the way he states that. Perhaps the need will not arise.

"Dr. Chang," I respond, "I believe immunotherapy has just gone on hold."

Good news travels fast, especially when I help it along. After giving thanks to God for this miracle in progress, I excitedly call Stan.

"This mental imagery of shutting off the blood supply to the tumors is really powerful," I say in awe. "It works."

"What do you mean?" Stan asks.

I recount the conversation with Dr. Chang, and can feel Stan's happiness over the phone.

"I'm going to be around for a long time," I say cheerily. "You had best get used to it."

"No problem," Stan replies. "Nothing would please me more."

My excitement continues to grow as I share the good news with my children, family and friends. Everyone I tell responds with an excitement that matches my own. And to further add to my happiness, the tubes are removed from my nose and throat, and I start on a soft diet consisting of liquids, Jell-O, and pudding. I can't possibly ask for anything more today.

Aside from fluid retention, and a temporary weight gain, I am healing well from the surgery. My use of pain medication is steadily decreasing. I have an appointment with Charles the day after I return home, for additional acupuncture treatments to alleviate pain, help reduce scarring and inflammation around the foot long incision, and strengthen my remaining kidney and weakened immune system. Marilyn is arriving from California this weekend to spend the first week with me at home. Her letter arrives with the afternoon mail.

> Dearest Sue,
>
> What a pain in the ass, abdomen and hip this all is. Surgery isn't any fun, but soon you'll be feeling much better, and I'll be there, so you can get me to wait on you, and maybe Stan will drop grapes in your mouth!!! And we'll all be celebrating your good health and speedy recovery. But you'd better watch out, because if you aren't nice to me, I'll hold a magnet up to your leg, and you won't be able to escape. Oh boy. This is just what I have been waiting for. Talk about co-dependency. Just think. Shortly I'll be there, and you'll wish you were back in the hospital with the cute male nurses.
>
> I love you,
> Marilyn

I put the card on my night stand, and laugh out loud. A week at home with Marilyn will be anything but dull.

The door to my room opens, and much to my delight, Kal and Karen walk in, arms loaded with gifts.

"You're early for my birthday," I laugh, hugging and kissing them both. "Right month, but wrong end of it."

"We wanted to make sure you had the latest in hospital wear," Karen says.

"After all," Kal adds, "we can't let you reflect poorly on the family."

I tear the wrapping paper off the large box. Nestled inside is a soft, feminine pajama set, and matching slippers.

"I'll bedazzle them now for sure," I comment.

"Save your bedazzling for me," Stan interjects.

"Is this the love struck guy?" Kal asks.

"The same," I answer.

Kal holds out his hand to Stan, and they shake.

"Let me really tell you about my sister," Kal begins earnestly.

"Kal, you're incorrigible. You would do that with all my boyfriends when you were just a kid," I laughingly exclaim.

"Yeah," Kal smiles. "And as I recall, you'd bribe me to shut up. So, what's it worth to you now, sis?"

"Behave yourself, Kal," Karen says playfully. "Don't scare Stan off. I like him."

"Okay," Kal agrees amicably, and changes the subject. "We brought someone to keep you company when Stan's not here. Someone else to snuggle with."

He hands me a smaller package. Inside is a soft and fuzzy stuffed pink rabbit.

"I love him," I say, cuddling the rabbit in my arms.

"Should I be jealous?" Stan asks impishly.

"Definitely. I have a thing for rabbits," I mischievously reply.

"What are you going to name him?" Karen interjects.

"I don't know," I answer. "I haven't thought about it."

"What's Dr. Chang's first name?" she persists.

"Alfred," I say.

"Alfie," Karen says. "It's perfect. Call him Alfie."

I laugh. "Alfie it is," I agree.

"And now for the piece-de-resistance," Kal states. "Knowing how much you love egg drop soup, we stopped at a Chinese restaurant, and bought some for you." He presents the large container with a flourish.

"Seems they didn't have plastic spoons," Karen continues, not missing a beat. "So what does your brother do? Ever so slowly, he backs up to a table, and quick as can be, drops a metal spoon into his pants.

"And here it is," Kal exclaims in a loud voice. Removing the spoon from his pants, he ceremoniously wipes it off, before handing it to me.

A YEAR OF MIRACLES

I laugh so hard my sides hurt. Looking around the room, I see Stan, Sharon, Elyssa, and Brent doubled over with laughter as well.

My hospital room stripped bare, looks institutional once again, as I wait with Stan and Marilyn for my discharge papers.

"I'm so glad to be getting out," I say, as Dr. Chang walks into the room.

"I just received the laboratory report," Dr. Chang begins. "It turned out exactly like the first one. Not a cancer cell to be seen."

"Thank God," I say, feeling blessed.

Marilyn, Stan, and I, beam at one another, and hug.

"I scheduled another liver biopsy ten days from now," Dr. Chang continues. "I still don't understand this."

"I will have the biopsy, but it's not going to show cancer," I say with heartfelt conviction.

"I hope so," Dr. Chang says. "I would like that."

"You'll see," I insist. "I just know it."

As Stan wheels me out of the hospital and into the waiting car, I look at my hospital discharge papers. Under patient diagnosis, renal cell carcinoma is written in bold print.

"You know," I say, waving the papers at Marilyn and Stan, "a time will come when that diagnosis no longer will apply to me."

CHAPTER 13

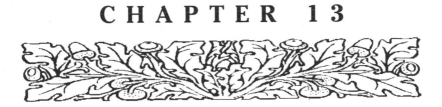

There is No False Hope

It is good to be home again, and to have Marilyn with me. Not just for her help in driving me to acupuncture appointments with Charles, and sessions with James. Not just for the shopping, cleaning, and cooking she cheerfully does. There is no doubt that I need assistance for now, but Marilyn's worth is measured in another infinitely more important way. The welcome home note I receive from her mother Evalyn states it clearly.

"I know that Marilyn's being with you will be a morale booster."

She is right.

"And as Indiana Jones says," her note continues in all earnestness, "May The Force Be With You."

And, It is.

The week Marilyn and I spend together helps strengthen not only my body, but also my spirit and soul. Sitting side by side, watching the Johnny Carson show, eyes glued to the television, we listen as Michael Landon, weaving together a mixture of wisdom, compassion and humor, speaks eloquently about his ongoing battle with pancreatic cancer. We sob noisily as Michael expresses intense love for his family, sharing how their love and strength, which he draws upon daily, comforts and sustains him. We put plastic straws in my nose when Stan stops by, to remind him of the night he professed his love, and howl with laughter at the look on his face. We meditate together lying on opposite ends of the sectional, giving ourselves over to healing visualizations. We talk late into the night, recounting the wild, zany adventures we have shared, and plan new ones. We explore both my fears and hers. No holds barred. Marilyn is positive and upbeat. She expects the best.

"I don't just believe in miracles," she fervently says. "I depend upon them."

As with all our time spent together, the days speed by, until all too soon Marilyn is gone, leaving me in a suddenly silent house. Why is it that the bad times seem to last forever, and the good times end too soon?

As the acupuncture sessions with Charles help alleviate the pain from surgery, and the anesthesia and morphine continue leaving my system, I begin to feel my body again. On good days this is a blessing, but on bad days, every ache and pain feels exaggerated, and leaves me wondering if the cancer is growing somewhere else. I know feeling this way is mostly due to nerves and fear, and being homebound for another week with too much time to think. Yet each time these feelings occur, they seem so very real. What I find most difficult is living with the uncertainty of not knowing if the cancer will recur. If it is completely gone. If my backache is anything more than a backache. If the outpatient liver biopsy scheduled for tomorrow will be benign as I believe it will, or cancerous as the doctors seem to expect. If. If. If. There are just too many ifs in my life. Still, my appetite is good, my strength is returning, and more days than not, I feel upbeat.

Susan is a dear, empathizing with me every time I turn to her with what I dub, "my being neurotic." She reminds me over and over, during my year long healing journey, that my fears are normal and will diminish in time. She is the one person I feel I can call on any hour of the day or night, for she has walked a similar path, and is most able to understand what I am experiencing. Listening to Susan's calm, steady voice, and loving words of wisdom and encouragement helps in comforting me. I am very thankful Susan is such an integral part of my life.

The liver biopsy is hell. There is no other way to state it. Dr. Chang is away at a conference for the day, and the doctors performing the biopsy, refuse to listen to me. I beg them to do a biopsy of the tumor that Dr. Chang didn't remove a portion of, but they are insistent on doing it their way.

"We are only thinking of your welfare," a smug faced doctor, condescendingly explains.

I am not a violent person, but I have a strong urge to punch that expression off his face.

"The second tumor is much more difficult and painful to get at. We will get the results we are looking for with a biopsy of the first, with considerably less pain to you," he concludes.

"The first tumor didn't show cancer, and it was tested twice," I argue. "That is why my doctor ordered another biopsy."

"Most likely, your doctor removed tissue around the tumor, and not a piece of the tumor itself," he insists, that same infuriating look on his face.

"It's not cancerous," I yell, losing my temper. "You are going to end up performing a biopsy of both tumors. My doctor is a top notch surgeon. I know he didn't mess up."

Finally, frustrated, enraged, and feeling totally discounted, I unwillingly give in.

A long needle is inserted through skin and bone, into my liver. I cannot be given anesthesia, and must lie quietly without moving. I howl in pain and outrage. The needle is withdrawn, and the cells are examined. I take deep, jagged breaths, dry my tears, and wait.

"We're going to do another needle aspiration into the tumor, and withdraw some more cells," the same doctor says, looking a little less smug.

"What did the first sample show?" I ask, eager to know.

"Just healthy cells," he answers sheepishly.

"I told you," I say triumphantly. "I'll let you do it one last time, and then I'm done."

The same procedure is repeated, with the same results.

"We need to do a needle aspiration on the other tumor." The doctor is now extremely uncomfortable as he speaks to me. All traces of smugness have vanished.

A YEAR OF MIRACLES

I consider it. I could insist on going home now, but I know Dr. Chang will want a biopsy of the other tumor, and I would only have to return at a later date.

"All right," I hesitatingly reply. "You can have a go at it twice, and then I'm out of here. I know my liver is cancer free."

The doctor is right about one thing though. Taking a needle aspiration of the second liver tumor makes the earlier procedure seem painless by comparison. Once again, the preliminary examination shows only healthy cells.

"I am dumbfounded," the doctor freely admits. "I haven't seen anything like this before. We will be doing additional laboratory work on the cells, but they certainly appear normal. There has to be some explanation for this."

"There is," I wholeheartedly agree. "But not a scientific one. It is a miracle from God."

A week passes waiting for the official results of the liver biopsy, to confirm what I know to be true, and officially learn through a phone conversation with Dr. Chang on a sunny May morning.

"Your liver is healthy and free of cancer, "Dr. Chang joyfully announces.

"Thank God," I fervently respond.

"This puts immunotherapy on hold indefinitely," Dr. Chang adds.

"I can live with that," I say gleefully. "What will happen next?"

"We will schedule you for a scan on July 3rd, and evaluate it from there," Dr. Chang responds.

"Meaning no immunotherapy, as long as the cancer doesn't recur," I say thoughtfully.

"Precisely," Dr. Chang replies.

I am becoming somewhat more comfortable living with this day in, day out uncertainty. I don't know if I will ever get used to it, and I strongly doubt that I will ever like it. On the plus side, I am finding this same uncertainty has positive value, for it is teaching me to cherish each day as a gift not to be taken for granted. I am experiencing life with a greater depth and breadth of emotions, and recognizing the miracles that define life more clearly than ever before. All told, I am learning some valuable lessons, no matter what the future may hold.

I am 51 today, and this birthday is a celebration of life, for I feel my life has been given back to me by God. I had thought no birthday would surpass my fiftieth, with the enormous birthday party I held to celebrate the beginning of the second half of my life. But I was wrong. When I turned fifty, I possessed only an intellectual understanding of my mortality, and still believed myself invincible. Now, knowing better, I am grateful to be alive. This past year has encompassed the best of times and the worst of times, and both have changed my life immeasurably. It was at my fiftieth birthday party that Stan entered my life. He has become such an integral, beloved part of my life, that I can barely remember a time when his presence was not constantly in my heart. He continues to teach me about love, and being a woman in the truest sense. The absolute trust I have in him, and in his love for me, strengthens my resolve to live life to the fullest. I am very hopeful as I begin this birthday year, that with God's intervention, the best will continue, while the worst will become a part of my past, and that the gifts from both will remain with me for however long I may live.

Stan arrives, a smile lighting his face. Kissing me soundly, he hands me a birthday card, and a small gift wrapped package. The sentiments expressed in the card brings tears to my eyes, and I sniffle audibly.

"Open the package," Stan eagerly says. "I can't wait any longer."

I tear off the wrapping paper, and open the velour box. Nestled within the satin lining is a stunning emerald ring.

"It's gorgeous," I manage to say, my voice choked with emotion. "I love it."

The emerald is so clear. It sparkles and catches the sunlight, as Stan lifts it from the box and slips it onto my finger.

A YEAR OF MIRACLES

"It's your birthstone," Stan says lovingly. "I give it to you as a symbol of my love."

I throw my arms around Stan, and kiss him passionately.

"I love it," I say happily. "Almost as much as I love you. I don't know how to thank you."

Stan grins. "Think about it," he says, his voice growing husky. "You're bound to figure it out."

That evening, after numerous birthday visits and calls from family and friends that reinforces my sense of being so deeply loved, I do a Runic Spread to gain an in-depth understanding of the coming year. I draw six Runes representing my foundation, my past, my present, my future, my challenge for the coming year, and the best possible outcome I can anticipate. Since a considerable amount of information is given, it requires some time to digest, contemplate and meditate on the spread. After noting the Runes I receive, I replace them in the bag, and draw a single Rune. This seventh Rune, the Rune of Resolution, gives me the essence of this next year of my life. It is the Rune of Joy and Light, and it is Reversed. It states:

> "Things are slow in coming to fruition. The process of birth is long and arduous, and fears arise for the safety of the "child" within. A crisis, a difficult passage... even if brief... is at hand. Consideration and deliberation are called for, because light and shadow are still intermixed and doubts and scruples might interfere with joyousness if not understood as timely to your growth. So stop your anxiety and ask yourself whether you posses the virtues of seriousness, sincerity, and emptiness. To possess them is to have tranquillity which is the ground for clarity, patience and perseverance.
>
> Seen in its true light, EVERYTHING IS A TEST. And so, focused in the present, sincere toward others, and trusting in your own process, know that you cannot fail."

THERE IS NO FALSE HOPE

It briefly crosses my mind as I read the Rune of Resolution, that the crisis at hand will be a recurrence of the cancer, but I immediately put that thought out of my mind, and focus instead on the last five words, "KNOW THAT YOU CANNOT FAIL."

Only one other thing remains for me to do. Cutting my horoscope for the year out of the newspaper, I tape it into my journal. It reads:

ON YOUR BIRTHDAY SUNDAY, MAY 26...
Loyal friends will open doors for you in the year ahead that you could never open on your own. Your wishes and desires can be realized through the good will you've established with key people.

That sounds good, I think. I am tired and content, happy, and grateful to be alive. I fall asleep easily, my cheek resting on the hand that now wears an emerald ring.

I am reading Bernie Seigel's book, when I come across a passage by a female cancer patient, who calls cancer, "the gift for the woman who has everything." Closing the book, I think about what I have just read. Though I don't yet agree with her, I think I understand what she means. My own journey with cancer has been, and continues to be, one of growth, transformation, and healing. I would not consciously choose cancer as a catalyst for growth, but in no way can I deny that is exactly what it has become for me. I am learning a great deal about myself. Some of it is difficult to learn, especially when I do not like what I discover. Still, every discovery is an opportunity to embrace the light, and move further away from the shadow side of my personality.

At my next appointment, I tell James that I am not a cancer personality as I define that, and James helps me look at my need for defining things. Historically, I have grown up letting my family, and the world at large, define me into who I know I am not, which makes it important now for me to define who

A YEAR OF MIRACLES

I know I am. With increasing awareness, I begin to recognize how I limit myself with definitions, and actually become less than I am. Using patience and perseverance, two qualities that don't come naturally to me, I am slowly transforming this constriction in my personality, as I journey beyond definition into becoming all that I can be.

My appointment to meet with Dr. Wicha, who I have chosen as my primary oncologist, is scheduled for June 3rd. When I enter his inner office, I am in for an unwelcome surprise. Dr. Wicha has been called out of town, and I learn I am to be seen by a colleague of his. Before I can object and reschedule the appointment, Dr. Arrogance enters the room. His manner is somewhat brusque and impersonal. He glances through my file, places it on the desk, and turns to me.

"When was your kidney removed?" he asks.

"April 30th," I reply.

"How has your recovery gone so far?" he prods.

"Really well. I grow stronger every day, and I'm beginning to feel like my old healthy self again," I say with pride.

Dr. Arrogance looks intently at me before he speaks once again.

"The cancer will return within a year. Every patient I know of with metastasized kidney cancer has had a recurrence within that time span."

He states it as a fact. In his mind, there are no exceptions.

I sit for a moment in disbelief, not trusting my ears.

"Immunotherapy is a promising new experimental treatment," Dr. Arrogance concludes. "It is your best hope."

I am so angry, so choked with rage, that words fail me. I stand up, and move woodenly toward the door. It is not until I am safely on the other side that my tears begin to flow.

I call James and Dr. Chang as soon as I can find a phone, and feel fortunate that they are both available to speak with me.

"It can't be true," I wail into the phone. "There have to be some people who don't have recurrences within a year."

"There are," they both assure me, sympathetic to my panic and pain. "It is not a hard and fast rule."

Stan, my children, and friends are besides themselves with anger.

"You have to do something," they urge me. "You just can't ignore this."

"I will talk with Dr. Wicha, as soon as he returns," I respond, feeling defensive.

Deep in my heart, I know that is not enough. The following day, feeling stronger and more capable, I write and send the following letter to Dr. Arrogance.

Dear Doctor Arrogance,

I met with you on June 3rd, in the hematology-oncology clinic, as Dr. Wicha was out of town that day. Although you may have intended to be helpful, I left the clinic angry and terribly upset. I felt you offered me little hope regarding my recovery from metastasized kidney cancer. You informed me that the cancer would return within a year... that every patient you knew of with metastasized kidney cancer has had a recurrence.

I am a highly educated, intelligent, informed woman, and I have done a considerable amount of reading about my disease. I know that many people experience recurrence, but you are the first and only physician who has told me point blank, "to expect it to recur." I would like to ask you, what gives you that right, or that infallible knowledge. Only God knows with absolute certainty what is in store for me. To state unequivocally that cancer will recur is a very destructive act. I came to my appointment feeling alive and hopeful, and left feeling angry and robbed of hope. Fortunately, I posses an overall positive attitude, a strong faith, and knowledge that nothing is set in stone... which has allowed me to regain my earlier state of mind. However, other patients may not possess this same ability, and may accept your words of pronouncement as a true fact of things to come, thereby losing hope, giving up, and ultimately proving you right.

I suggest you familiarize yourself with two books by Bernie Siegel, M.D.. They are "Love, Medicine and Miracles," and "Peace, Love, and Healing." Dr. Siegel is a surgeon at Yale Hospital, and works extensively with cancer patients. To quote Dr. Siegel,

"What you have to understand is that there is a biology of the individual as well as a biology of the disease, each affecting the other. On the day of diagnosis, we don't know either well enough to use a pathology report to predict the future."

And to quote him once more,

"If I'm accused of offering false hope, my answer is that there is no false hope… only false no hope… because we don't know the future for an individual."

I believe your intent as a physician is to help, but in saying what you said to me, you missed the mark. Please think about how you say what you say to individuals with cancer, and leave them with their hope intact. It can't hurt, and it certainly can help.

P.S., Dr. Wicha is familiar with the work of Dr. Siegel, if you would like to discuss these books with a colleague.

I feel increasingly better, as I write, post, and mail the letter to Dr. Arrogance. My desire to help educate the medical profession in this arena is off to a running start, despite the fact that Dr. Arrogance will neither acknowledge nor respond to my letter.

THERE IS NO FALSE HOPE

The following week I am in Los Angeles, attending a weekend seminar with Marilyn entitled "The Alchemy of Adversity." It is being presented by Lazaris, a non-physical entity, who is channeled by Jach Pursell. Despite my hesitation to make the long four and a half hour flight so soon after two major surgeries, my desire to be at the seminar overcomes my initial caution. I can always catch up on my rest later, I reason, and this opportunity may not present itself again. The seminar turns out to be everything I had hoped for and more. In addition to the sheer joy of being in the presence of Lazaris, I learn about many unhealthy beliefs and patterns that help promote disease, which I have been unaware of. Better yet, Lazaris teaches several powerful techniques and meditations to help change them into healthy forms of expression. And as always, there is that priceless gift of spending a whole week at the ocean with Marilyn. As we take our daily walks along the beach, I find myself reveling in both the sun on my skin and our time spent together.

I am surprised to awaken one morning a few days after the seminar feeling frightened. The sore back I am experiencing has refueled my fear of recurrence. I decide to work with one of the techniques I have learned at the seminar, and enter a meditation where my worst fear of recurrence is realized. As I do, I experience all the attendant emotions. Finally, as I have been taught, I call in both my Higher Self for guidance and support, and my Future Self for courage. My Future Self acknowledges her healing accelerated as her faith and trust in God's love and desire for her to be whole grew. My sore back is just a sore back she says, for I have over-extended myself physically. She suggests a technique in which I become very small, and climb down my ribs and vertebrae one by one, soothing and massaging them. As a final step, I sprinkle magical healing powder on them so they have the sparkle of vitality and good health.

My Future Self informs me she is sixty years old, though she looks much younger, and has been happily married to Stan for eight years. She has written a very successful book on healing from cancer, which has helped many people, is a sought after inspirational speaker, and works with people with life threatening illness. She is also a talented amateur photographer, who especially delights in taking pictures of her grandchildren. She and Stan travel frequently, both for business and pleasure. She is very happy, very spiritual, and very much alive.

I come out of meditation believing I am healthy, and knowing I have found a way of working with and releasing this fear whenever it recurs. I decide to repeat this meditation several times during the next few days, whether or not the fear is present. My goal is to integrate this meditation into my very being, thereby strengthening and fortifying my ability to handle this pervasive fear. After giving thanks, I find myself feeling serene, and imbued with a sense of well being. It is a fitting way to begin my last full day in California with Marilyn.

Back home, I agree to a joint presentation with James, for the enlightenment of the medical community of doctors, nurses, and mental health professionals on "Adjunctive Cancer Treatments." James will do his presentation, and then I will speak about my experiences, both traditional and alternative, and the healing that has taken place. I am very excited about this, despite my apparent lack of success with Dr. Arrogance. I believe it is crucial that the medical community recognize and respect the individual with cancer as an active participant in his or her own treatment and healing process, even when this includes choosing therapies that go beyond radiation, chemotherapy, and surgery. It is equally crucial for the individual with cancer to know, to believe, and to fight for her or his right to choose adjunctive cancer therapies alongside mainstream ones, even when one's physician is less than enthused with that choice. And it is imperative for both to remember, that the "individual with cancer" is first and foremost a unique, living, breathing, feeling, thinking, human being, who happens to have a disease called cancer, but is so much more than that disease.

The presentation goes well, and I feel comfortable being a part of it. Some of the participants commend me, saying I am courageous to speak about my experiences, but I don't view it as an act of courage. I have only shared that which I am comfortable sharing. Besides, having Sharon and Susan present in the audience has made it that much easier to do.

After the presentation, there is a question and answer period. A young doctor questions me closely about living with false hope. I ask him to explain what he means.

"Wouldn't it be more difficult If you believed you were not going to have a recurrence, and then had one, then to know from the start that you are likely to have a recurrence?" he asks. "And isn't it my duty to tell you the truth?"

"Even though I believe I won't have a recurrence, I know the possibility always exists," I slowly answer, feeling my way. "But with my belief, I live each day fully, expecting the best. If I believed I was likely to have a recurrence, I would live each day in fear, waiting and watching for signals to let me know the cancer has returned. No one knows that there will be a tomorrow, but we all believe there will, and plan for it. I don't want you or anyone else to take that away from me."

"But isn't it my duty to tell you the truth?" he persists.

"What is the truth?" I ask, as he meets my gaze.

"That a cancer like yours is considered terminal," he replies in obvious discomfort.

"Have people survived my kind of cancer?" I ask softly.

"Hardly any, just a tiny handful," he answers, his discomfort level increasing.

"Then tell me that some people have survived this type of cancer," I fire back, "and that I could be one of them. You aren't promising me I will be, but you aren't taking my hope away. In fact, you are giving me the hope I just might need, to be the next in that tiny handful of survivors."

"Thank you," he responds thoughtfully. "I can see your point."

"Thank you also," I say, moved. "You don't know how much you have brightened my day."

As July 3rd draws closer, though I do all I know to remain calm, centered, and trusting, I am frightened. Two days before my scan, Michael Landon dies from pancreatic cancer.

A YEAR OF MIRACLES

Although I am only one of many who love him and pray for his recovery, I have felt an extra special bond with Michael since the day I learned about my own cancer diagnosis, which was also the day I learned of his. Now barely three months later, Michael is dead, a terrifying reminder of how quickly cancer can destroy a life. It does not help to learn the following day of Lee Remick's death from kidney cancer, after a courageous two and a half year battle. That both these fine souls died with dignity and as an inspiration to millions is not lost on me. I hear the voices of loved ones telling me what an inspiration I am for them. I would not choose to be this kind of inspiration, but then again, who would? I remind myself that the first post-operative scan has to be the scariest, and that with time they will become less problematical. At any rate, I hope that will be the case, for I plan on being around for many more years to come.

The night before the scan, Stan tells me just how much I mean to him.

"I don't even want to contemplate what life would be like without you," he says fervently.

"Are you nervous about my scan?" I ask quietly.

"A little," he acknowledges sheepishly, "even though I believe you are fine."

"Me too," I quickly agree, "but I'm still also nervous."

"Because of you, I no longer feel alone," Stan admits in a hushed voice. "These last few years, I have experienced wave after wave of pain, as the people I love most fall ill."

"I can only imagine," I murmur.

"First Lynne. And now both my mother and father are seriously ill, and I feel so helpless," Stan says in a grief stricken voice. "I throw myself into my work as a way to cope and gain some distance, but it doesn't work all that well."

"And now me," I add sadly.

"Yes, that's true," Stan responds, "but you are different. You are going to live. You are not going to be another loss in my life."

"No loss," I agree hugging him with all my might. "You've got me babe, and I'm coming through this a winner."

THERE IS NO FALSE HOPE

I am relatively relaxed the actual day of the scan. Feeling God is with me, I have absolute faith and trust I am healthy, until the radiologist decides to take some additional x-rays to check behind my esophagus. Suddenly, my faith, my trust, and God appear to desert me, and I am thrown into a full blown panic attack. Even after the radiologist informs me there most likely is nothing to be concerned about, I am not reassured. My logical, rational mind agrees, but my fear is stronger than logic. With the unexpected loss of my faith, my trust, and my connection to God, the dark demons of my shadow side run rampant once more.

Because of the holiday weekend, I will not learn the results for a few days, and I find myself wondering how I will make it through the agonizing wait. What disturbs me the most is how easily my faith and trust in both God and my healing has abandoned me, and I am deeply saddened by this realization. I sense this as a turning point in my spiritual life. Recognizing my faith and trust in God is not as strong as I believed it to be, areas where I still need to work are revealed. It is not as if I have consciously lied to myself, for I honestly believed myself stronger than I am. Spending the next two days in prayer and meditation, I ask God's help in regaining my faith and trust. God is patient and loving, leading me to insights that help strengthen my belief in a positive outcome.

By the following morning, I am at peace with myself once again, trusting that all will be well, and able to wait for the official report. As soon as I achieve that degree of serenity the phone rings. It is Dr. Chang, who calmly informs me the scan shows no signs of cancer. We schedule the next scan for early September. I hope to progress far enough by then, to go through the scan with my faith and trust intact. Feeling the healing love of God with me once again, I celebrate freedom from fear with my own internal fireworks.

CHAPTER 14

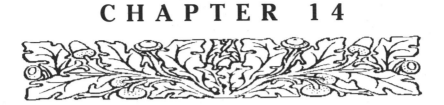

Personal Best

I learn the Washtenaw County American Cancer Society is seeking volunteers to drive cancer patients to their radiation and chemotherapy appointments. I am driving again, feeling healthy, still off from work, and filled with gratitude at being alive. With more than a little free time to spare, I call and volunteer my services. My schedule is flexible, but I usually drive two mornings a week. As I get to know the men and women I transport, and talk about my own recent experience with cancer, I see the light of hope shine brighter in many eyes. For now, this is my way of working with cancer patients that fits within my own comfort level. Still enmeshed in my recent experience as a cancer patient, I lack the necessary perspective which would enable me to work with other cancer patients on a deeper, more intense level. Though I am certain that such a time resides somewhere in my future, I know better than to try to force it now. In the meantime, living in the present, I give what I can, when I can.

Elyssa stops by during her lunch hour several times a week, to chat and share a meal together. Sometimes, I will fix lunch for the two of us, and other times she will surprise me with wonderful sandwiches from Zingerman's. It is a ritual she performed almost daily during my stay in the hospital, nurturing me with delicious food, while rescuing me from mediocre hospital fare. We talk about everything and anything. It is a pleasure to be able to laugh wholeheartedly, relax, and dream together. The long, lazy summer days pass with fewer extremes of highs and lows than the rollercoaster days of spring. I feel myself unwinding, and shared afternoon lunches with Elyssa contribute to this delightful mellowing out.

Riding in "Morph," a 19 foot Airstream RV, the rain sketching patterns on the windowpane, Stan as close as a heartbeat away, we begin a two week adventure that will take us into Maine, New Hampshire, and Vermont. In Ohio, the sun breaks free of the clouds, and a double rainbow spreads across the sky, remaining within view for many minutes. Evening falls, and as we drive into the night under a cloak of darkness we talk about matters of life and death. Shadow intermingles with light as I turn to study Stan's face, and I feel a flood of desire wash over me. Hours later, snug on our featherbed, we slowly, tenderly, make love. Drifting off to sleep on a balmy August night, safe in the arms of the one I love, I know all is well in my world.

We are an hour outside of Philadelphia, heading toward Stan's childhood home, to visit his parents, who are elderly and sick. The closer we get, the more troubled a look Stan wears on his face, and I sense we are headed toward a disaster zone. My own nervousness about our first meeting quickly fades, as my desire to put a smile back into Stan's strained eyes grows stronger with each passing mile. I close my eyes, and pray to God for guidance and strength.

I don't realize how difficult this part will be for me, until I do it. Arriving at the Fox Chase Cancer Center with Stan and his parents, we wait for his father to be readmitted. Memories, much closer to the surface than I am aware of, come fast and furious. I speak with Stan's father Jesse about the importance of living with hope. He holds my left hand in his, while gently running his right hand through my hair. He listens closely, looks deeply into my eyes, smiles sadly, but doesn't utter a word. While Stan is escorting his father to his room, I go outdoors to walk in the cancer survivors garden. A large tree beckons to me, and as I lean against its warm, smooth bark, I am filled with a deep sense of peace. Despite being quite certain that Jesse and I will not meet again, I feel we have connected on a deep soul level today.

We stop overnight in New Jersey to visit my childhood friend Sheila, her husband George, a cancer survivor for over twenty years, their daughter Betsy, Sheila's sister Alice, her husband and two young sons, and their widowed mother Lucy. It is wonderful to see them again. My mother and Lucy had been the closest of friends from childhood on, as have Sheila and I. The whole family likes Stan, and makes him feel immediately welcome. During breakfast, as I cut an East Coast bagel, Stan matter-of-factly states that his first wife cut bagels the same way. It is the first time I have heard Stan refer to Lynne as his first wife, and he seems to realize this as soon as the words leave his mouth. I laughingly ask Stan how many wives he has not told me about, but the significance of the remark is not lost on me. Nor is it lost on Sheila, as I later learn.

I love Maine, especially Arcadia National Park, with its craggy coastline and wonderful huge red boulders sprayed by the crashing surf. I delight in the time I spend lying on smooth, inviting, wet rocks warmed by the sun, listening to the ocean and the song of the seagulls, the breeze refreshing and soft on my skin, with Stan just an arm's length away. Another day, we go on a whale watching expedition. It is cold and windy at sea, and I am glad for my down parka as I stand on the deck, the spray wetting my face and my clothing. The ocean is teeming with life. Whales, porpoises and seals frolic nearby. An unexpected gust of wind abducts Stan's bright orange cap, and sends it spinning wildly overboard. We laugh thinking of some gentle giant of the sea surfacing with an orange cap on its tail or fin.

Part of our vacation is spent hunting minerals, in "off the beaten path" rock shops. Other days we dig for them in the quarries that abound. Morph is rapidly gaining weight as our collection grows, but pal that he is, he humors us, and seldom complains. Just grunts and sputters some as he transports us uphill. Ours must truly be a match made in heaven, because I can't think of too many other people, who can pass the evenings "scrubbing rocks" in complete and mutual ecstasy.

A YEAR OF MIRACLES

August 30th, exactly four months since kidney surgery, we hike the White Mountains of New Hampshire. The gorgeous late summer day dawns warm and sunny, as we begin our eight mile round trip trek to Carter Notch Hut, on the Appalachian Trail. The guide book states the average hiking time as six hours, and rates the difficulty of the trail as moderate. As morning turns into afternoon, I come to the belief the book is geared toward Olympic hikers. The trail is extremely rugged. Climbing over the huge boulders that make up the trail is hard work. Finally we reach the hut, view the pristine cobalt blue lake in the mountain, refresh ourselves with lemonade, and start working our way back down, climbing those same treacherous boulders. It is more strenuous going up, but much trickier getting down.

At times I wonder if I will make it. I am more cautious than before the hip replacement as to how and where I place my feet on the steep ascent and descent. Stan offers to help me, but I am insistent on doing this myself. Initially, I am angry, frustrated, and self critical of my physical limitations. I want my old body back. And though I wish I was above it, I am also envious Stan has no limitations. As I continue to persevere, making it past each obstacle, I realize how blessed I am to have progressed this far. Drenched in sweat and breathing heavily, I begin to feel a real sense of pride in this physical accomplishment. There are many people, both younger and older than me, without physical limitations, who lack the stamina to hike this trail. By the time we reach the parking lot and the comforts of Morph, my body feels sore and tired; a condition which will prove only temporary. But the challenges met and overcome on this hike will remain permanently etched in my mind. Willingly, I give myself over to experiencing the incredible high of having done my personal best.

Outside of Buffalo, New York, the breathtaking views of New England but a sweet memory, we drive through flat countryside on our final lap to Ann Arbor, a place I have not thought of these past sixteen days. I am returning for a CAT scan which I expect to go well, but still feel uneasy about, and to my own home where Stan is a frequent visitor, but does not yet reside. Having quickly grown accustomed to days and nights spent together, I don't look forward to the change in our living arrangements. I am feeling more of a desire for the kind of commitment that will join our lives together, and allow us to create a home of our own. I know that is impossible for a numbers of reasons, not the least of which involves Stan's twenty one year old daughter Natalie, who is devoted to her mother's memory, presently lives at home, and is less than happy about our relationship. It is fitting that it will soon be Labor Day, for the changes I am being driven toward feel laborious.

I am barely a veteran of one post operative CAT scan, and although I believe they will become easier with the passage of time, I am light years away from feeling at ease. Hopefully, some not too distant day, that will no longer be true. Assuredly, this continual movement toward serenity, clarity, balance, trust, and faith, no matter how frightening the circumstances, is a vision that I hold dear. My Higher Self lives there. My human self still has a way to go. This is only my second post operative scan, and despite the scan going smoothly, I feel agitated and anxious. Due to a longer than usual wait for results because of another long holiday weekend, I promise myself this is the last scan I will schedule during a holiday. This is a promise I will not break, for it is essential to treat myself with kindness and gentleness, and not create more difficulties than already exist. I manage to get through the long wait, secluding myself for extended periods of prayer and meditation. Rosh Hashanah, which is the start of the Jewish New Year, I learn all is well. I am ecstatic that the good news arrives on this High Holy Day. Taking this as a sign from God that this will be a year of good health, I gratefully give thanks.

Mid September, I receive permission to return to work on a half time basis. My clients, eager to see me after a six months absence, happily welcome me back. I pace myself, making certain to not overwork, thankful for the monthly disability check which allows me this luxury. The first week back, four new clients phone wanting to see me, and I recognize the Universe is supportive of my return to work. Since my continued health and well being is of primary importance, and I am committed to attending to them, I accept two clients, and refer the other two to Pat. Slowly, but surely, I am learning to set limits, and take better care of myself.

In early October, Stan and I leave for a long camping weekend up north, where we anticipate seeing the colors turn. Fall in Michigan is breathtaking, as the leaves on the trees turn red, orange, and gold. Although winter is not far behind, it is sunny, mild and quite spectacular right now.

This weekend will mark a major turning point in our relationship. Saturday evening, as we sit around a blazing campfire roasting marshmallows, Stan confides how unexpectedly our relationship evolved for him.

"I thought I would date for some time before finding a woman I wanted to be with," Stan hesitatingly admits.

I sit very still, heart beating wildly, listening intently.

"Our relationship isn't one that I consciously chose. That our friendship turned romantic, surprised and delighted me." Stan falls silent for a moment, takes a deep breath and determinedly continues. "The fantasy I had of dating other women is still with me, and I wonder if down the road I will regret not having lived it out."

I am stunned by his honesty. We have been through so much together, as friends and lovers. Sixteen months to be exact. What does he want now?

"Do you want to date other women?" I ask, grateful for the darkness of the night.

"No, I don't, and I don't want you to date either," he unhesitatingly answers. "I just want to talk about it, because I see myself closing doors on an area of my life I thought I would be exploring."

I realize that I have consciously chosen to be involved with Stan, whereas for him it was "something that just happened," and evolved from there.

"Sometimes, when we close one door we open another door that has even more to offer," I slowly respond. "What we have together is so very special."

"Is it really?" Stan is completely sincere in his asking.

"What do you think?" Tears roll down my cheek, and I turn my face away.

"I don't know," Stan quietly answers. "My only other relationship was with Lynne, and it was different than ours, but also loving and quite wonderful."

"Stan, you are so very blessed. Few people experience this kind of bond, and God has bestowed it upon you twice. It's no wonder you don't realize how special it is. It's all you have ever known, so you take it for granted. It might help to look at other relationships, study them, and then see what you think." Not knowing what else to say, I fall silent.

"Thank you," Stan says with obvious relief.

"For what?" I ask confused.

"For being you. For not getting angry with me. For talking about this, even though I know it has to be difficult for you."

I turn towards Stan. He puts his arm around me, and I rest my head on his shoulder. I am certain everything will work out for the best. There is no doubt in my heart, that our finding each other is a gift from God.

"Our relationship has changed for the better," Stan says playfully the following week. "I thought you might like to know that."

"What do you mean?" I ask puzzled.

Stan takes my hands in his, and looks at me lovingly. "I consciously choose to be with you Susan, in love and in joy, knowing that God is blessing our union."

I nod my agreement, too overcome with emotion to immediately speak.

As the weeks go by, I can sense the difference in our relationship. We grow even closer. Stan shares more of himself with me, and being apart is difficult. We spend time together as often as we can, and I literally feel my heart expanding in love. I think myself the luckiest woman on the face of the earth, and am aware of smiling and laughing more often than not.

I begin "Writing From The Right Side Of The Brain," a creative writing class I have taken many times before, taught by Kay Gould Caskey and Jim Johnson, who have become my friends. I love the class, the way it is run, and the innate creativity that flows through the group. Each time I participate I grow as a writer, which brings pleasure and a sense of pride. One evening prior to leaving, we are given an assignment for the following week.

"Find an old photograph of someone you know," Kay says, "and write a story about the photograph."

At home, I eagerly leaf through an old photograph album. It is filled with pictures of my grandparents, mother, uncle, aunt, and relatives I never knew who died in the Holocaust. I find a photograph of my mother as a young woman, sitting in a 1930 Ford. It is a picture I love, and one I have looked at many times during my childhood. I place it in front of me, and begin to write.

The Woman in The 1930 Ford

A young woman leans out the passenger window of a 1930 Ford. Her arms are demurely crossed, and her chin rests gracefully on her hands. Her wavy auburn shoulder length hair is swept to one side, lending an air of sensual abandonment to an otherwise angelic face. Behind her rise the tall stately brownstones with small, square, never-ending panes of glass, wide inviting steps, and marble urns overflowing with summer flowers. She has lived on this street since she was seven, and knows its secrets well. If you were to look closely, you would see dried tears alongside the brilliant smile that masks her pain. Her heart has recently been broken. She tells no one, but on an entry dated August, 1934 she has written across the back of the photograph:

"To the sweet and tender memories he once brought to my heart. In the summer of 1934, I experienced a great love and a constant yearning for the one I thought I could love forever, but as all good things come to an end, this one had to go through the usual preliminaries. I am not sorry to have experienced this feeling so commonly called love."

His name is Teddy. He is tall, handsome, and wealthy. He is a law student at Columbia University. Her name is Miriam. She is petite, beautiful, and middle class. She works as a secretary and takes night classes at N.Y.U. He can trace his family history back to the early 1800's when his great great grandfather first set foot on American soil, changed his name from Liebowitz to Lee, and set about removing all traces of his Jewish heritage. Her family immigrated from Russia when she was seven, attends synagogue religiously, and the preferred spoken language in her home is Yiddish. His family thinks she is beneath him, and orders that he give her up. When he refuses, his family threatens to disown him. She never knows what could have been, for Teddy does not fight for love. She is left with only memories.

She does not know it now, but she will meet another man. His name will be Daniel. He will be of similar background, arriving from Russia two months before his birth, becoming the first child in his family to be born in America. For this, he will be pampered and spoiled by parents, grandparents, uncles and aunts. He will be taught that he can do no wrong, and he will grow to believe it. This lesson will ruin her life, destroy their marriage, and scar the two children born of this union. The love will be gone long before he is, and her memories will be bitter.

She will raise her children alone, and never remarry. She will be the kind of mother her children adore, for she will pour her love into them. It will not be until they are adults, that they will begin to question her choices. She will spend the last twenty eight years of her life never loving or being loved by a man. If she misses it, she will never speak of it. If she cries at night from loneliness, her children will never know. She will joyously welcome grand-parenthood. Her grandchildren's first three words will be, mama, dada, and nana, and they will love her dearly.

In the winter of 1974, she will awaken on too many days feeling ill. She will be frightened, but will tell no one, until she can no longer bear the pain. She will be admitted to the hospital for tests, and will be diagnosed with pancreatic cancer. She will survive surgery, only to die five months later, two weeks shy of her sixty first birthday. Her family will grieve her death, but will be comforted by the loving memories they hold of her in their hearts. Many years later, her daughter will come across a photograph of a young woman, leaning out the window of a 1930 Ford, and will write about her mother.

As I reread what I have written, I am shaken to the core. That my mother lovingly gave so much of herself to others, yet asked so little for herself, saddens me deeply. My kind and gentle mother believed in me, taught me to believe in myself, and to aim for the best in life. How I wish she had lived the life she taught me to strive for, and that it had included the love of a good man, who would have cherished her "in sickness and in health."

James finishes reading the piece about my mother, and looks at me thoughtfully.

"Just as kidney cancer is emotionally related to what we hold on to, and what we let go of, and breast cancer to nurturance issues, pancreatic cancer deals with stoicism," he states. "Your mother appears to have been a very stoic woman."

"How would you describe stoic?" I ask.

"Someone who outwardly appears unemotional and unconcerned about the tragedies and losses in their life. Someone who may inwardly be in great pain, but doesn't show it, or share it," he responds.

My mind runs backwards as it reviews my childhood and early adulthood with my mother. Except for a few occasions, James' assessment is right.

"She wasn't stoic when Kal or I experienced pain. She was loving and comforting," I say. "Just stoic around her own pain, and that was beginning to change. She was more openly sharing her last few years."

"Your mother was evolving both spiritually and psychologically." James pauses and then resumes. "Who knows what would have happened, had she lived."

"I miss her, but I often feel her presence. Especially since being diagnosed with cancer. And I can still feel her belief in me," I say in a clear, strong voice.

"She's your mother, and she very much wants you to live. She wants you to have what she never had." James falls silent.

"I know," I say, my voice filling with emotion. "That's just the way my mother is."

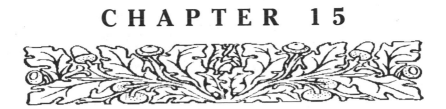

CHAPTER 15

Recurrence

Each time I have a CAT scan, I learn a lesson about faith and trust in a slightly different form. This time, I think my faith and trust are unshakable, but I am wrong. I am well prepared for the scan, through weeks of prayer and meditation. I look and feel great, and expect the scan to reflect that. On November 4, 1991, Susan once again accompanies me to the hospital. Having had breast cancer ten years earlier and completely recovered, Susan is all too familiar with the emotions that can erupt when facing a scan. Now, as a cancer victor, who has walked her talk, she is consistently available to help me through these trying times. I find having Susan with me during those times when any and all of my fears can be instantaneously triggered, both comforting and reassuring. My appreciation runs much deeper than my words can convey.

I am in control of myself as I lay on the table following instructions to take a deep breath, hold it, and let it out again, as the machine takes endless pictures of my abdomen and chest. I am in control of myself as the radiologist reads the pictures, and I lay watching through the window that separates us.

I am in control as I ask the technician why the doctor wants to take additional pictures, and she replies, "I just follow orders. I don't ask questions."

I feel my control slipping as another technician enters the room, and says, "the doctor wants more pictures."

"I'm starting to feel concerned," I say, watching my serenity crumble. "I want to know what is going on."

"It's nothing to worry about," the second technician assures me. "It's only a technical problem. The solution we injected into your veins didn't move into your bowels, so we are retaking the pictures, hoping the dye will move down. It happens all the time."

"What if it doesn't move?" I ask pensively.

"Then you get to go home. The pictures will be checked against your last scan, to make sure everything lines up."

"Is it not going down because of a blockage?" I ask, feeling on edge .

"There's no blockage," he replies gently. "I wouldn't worry about it."

"Of course you wouldn't," I think. "You probably haven't had to deal with cancer."

"How do the rest of the pictures look?" I ask cautiously.

"They look good," he answers, and smiles at me.

"Are you telling me the truth?"

"Why would I lie to you?" he replies, puzzled.

"You wouldn't," I answer, and mean it.

Pictures taken, I get down from the table, and walk to the dressing room, where I change into my clothes. I talk with Susan about what has occurred.

"I mostly held onto my faith and trust," I tell her. "Even when I was feeling scared. Even when I was questioning, I didn't lose my faith and trust."

I am feeling proud of myself. Susan, as always, is being Susan; very loving and supportive. We leave the hospital and stop at Angelo's for lunch.

"It's my treat," I insist, feeling expansive.

Afterwards, I drive Susan to work.

It isn't until early evening that I have a delayed reaction. My stomach turns queasy. I feel nauseous. Doubts start creeping into my mind. I have a bad feeling about this scan. I obsess. I do the Lazaris worst case scenario. I pray. I meditate. It doesn't dissolve my fear. I turn to the Runes and the Medicine Cards. The messages tell me to have faith. It will all work out for the best.

I feel like I don't have eyes to see, or ears to hear, and that I am using my strength against myself. Not knowing what else to do, I go to sleep. The bad feeling goes along with me.

I awaken in the morning praying my faith is stronger than my fear. I shower, dress, and go to work. Work takes my mind off the fear, but when I return home, it returns. I dial the phone and talk with Susan.

"I'm just being neurotic, but humor me," I say. "I need your help."

Susan gently reminds me that I am less fearful than I was the past two times, while I waited for results. I think about that, and realize it is true. I try taking comfort from that realization, but the bad feeling won't go away. Once again, I turn to the Medicine Cards.

"What is it I need to learn while waiting for the result of the scan?" I ask reverently.

I draw Bear Reversed. Its message reads:

> "Your internal dialogue has confused your perception of your truths. In seeking answers from others, you have placed your own knowing aside. The time has come to regain your authority, for no one knows better than you, what is timely and proper for your evolution. Reclaim the power of knowing. Allow the thoughts of confusion to be laid to rest as clarity emerges. To know yourself, is to know your body, your mind, and your spirit. Use your strengths to overcome your weaknesses, and know that both are necessary to your evolution. Journey with Bear to the quietness of your cave, and hibernate in silence. Dream your dreams and own them. Then in strength you will be ready to discover the honey waiting in the Tree of Life."

I feel a new strength emerging. In my deepest of hearts, I am healthy and free of cancer. I have faith in God's love for me. I believe God's Will is for me to prosper and thrive. I am not completely free of the bad feeling, but my trust in what I know to be true for me is growing stronger. I am doing the very best I can today. Tomorrow, I will search for the honey.

The following day, I am in session, when the answering machine picks up the call from Dr. Chang. A sense of foreboding settles in my chest, as I excuse myself and rush to the phone.

"Susan," Dr. Chang says, sadness thickening his voice, "there is the start of tumor re-growth on your seventh rib."

"No," I scream silently. "No! No! No!"

"Oh, Dr. Chang," I say, completely devastated, "this isn't what I at all expected, or ever wanted to hear."

"Nor is it what I want to be telling you," he says in a solemn voice, "but, unfortunately, it is what the scan shows. It appears radiation temporarily suppressed the cancer cells, and now they are multiplying again."

I have known from the start that recurrence was a real possibility, and that radiation is seldom effective against kidney cancer. But I have convinced myself otherwise over these past six months, and fully believed I would be the exception.

"What do we do now?" I ask dully.

"We treat you as we had planned," Dr. Chang answers. "The good news is that the cancer has not spread anywhere else in your body. The tumor is very small, and is relatively slow growing. You are in good health, and an overall excellent candidate for the experimental immunotherapy that we previously discussed. That is, if you still agree on treating it that way."

"What other options do I have?"

"You could look into additional radiation, although I wouldn't recommend that avenue."

"No," I say in a strangled voice. "It doesn't work. I don't want to do that."

"There is interferon therapy, which is not as powerful or successful."

"No," I say grief thickening my words. "I want the best."

"Then we're looking at Interleukin 2 and immunotherapy," he responds.

"All right," I agree, straining to hear his words through the thick fog that surrounds me. "Let's do it. Let's get rid of that sucker."

We talk about beginning the process the following week, and arrange a date and time. I hang up the phone, too stunned to feel anything. I have totally shut off my emotions, and am operating on automatic pilot. I go back to my client, and complete the session, growing more numb, and going deeper into shock with each passing minute.

I find myself home a few hours later, though I have no recollection of driving there. Alternating between disbelief, shock, fear, sadness, and anger, I move woodenly around the house, my mind racing ahead. I know I will need to tell Stan, my children, my family, and friends once again, and I dread it. I don't want to add pain to the lives of the people I love most, yet there is no way to spare them. More than ever, I need their belief in my ability to heal from this recurrence. But how can I ask them to believe in something that I myself don't believe in right now?

I am so mad at God. How can I keep my faith and trust in God's mysterious ways, when I feel totally betrayed and abandoned by God? I have worked so hard and long on keeping my faith and trust intact, and for what? Why did God let this happen to me again? What is God planning for me now? Doesn't God love me anymore? It will take some time before I come to terms with the feelings I am experiencing now, and regain my faith and trust in God's love for me. I will eventually recognize that there is a purpose in all God does, and when one door closes, God opens a new door that has even more to offer. These are the exact words I spoke so easily to Stan that October night around our campfire. It will take this terrifying turn of events before I really walk my talk, and make those words ring true for me.

Stan is stunned by the news, and I watch as his face crumbles. We cling to one another and sob, until our river of tears finally abates. Exhausted, and overwhelmed by grief, we woodenly crawl into bed. Still holding each other, desperately seeking a comfort and warmth that is not to be found, we lie locked together in pain. Stan is fortunate, for he is able to fall asleep, but sleep eludes me. I lie in bed absolutely convinced I am going to die. There is not the slightest doubt in my mind of the final outcome. I feel completely helpless and overcome by despair. I lie awake for hours as Stan sleeps, and watch as all my hopes and dreams turn to dust. I make lists in my mind, and divide my possessions among my children. I write letters to each one of them, to be opened after my death. I think about the kind of funeral I want, and decide it should be a celebration of my life. I debate whether or not to be an organ donor, and can't reach a decision. Finally, as the sun begins to rise, I sleep.

I am in James' office sobbing, hysterical, and raving like a lunatic. I am out of control and quite overwrought. James sits quietly in his chair, looking at me lovingly. I feel his warmth and serenity, and finally fall silent.

"You don't have to die," he says soothingly. "You can live. I can help you."

I relax some, and listen to James' words.

"You've experienced a great shock, and you're reacting to it emotionally. That is quite natural and understandable. But remember Susan, you are a fighter, and you can influence the outcome," he says calmly. "Once you can accept that the cancer has recurred, your natural optimism and positive attitude will soon return, along with your determination to do everything in your power to live."

"I want to live. More strongly than ever. But I'm afraid I'm going to die," I wail, tears welling up.

"You might die," James factually responds, "and you might live. There are never those kind of guarantees in life. But since you are alive, please decide on something that is very important. Where do you want to focus your energies now?"

"On living." The words come flying out of my mouth.

"Good," James says, looking pleased. "Let's do just that. For starters, I would encourage you to postpone immunotherapy for three months."

I start to protest, but James silences me.

"I will speak with Dr. Chang," he reassures me, "and make certain that it is a feasible plan. I believe it will be, because the tumor is very small and slow growing, and three months shouldn't make much of a difference."

"But it can grow and spread," I interject, apprehensively.

"There is a small risk of that," he agrees, "but I think the time you can buy will be more than worth the risk. And remember Susan, you will be working with the technique you learned, to try to dissolve this tumor. The same one you used so successfully on dissolving your liver tumors. And don't forget, you will be having regular scans during these three months. So if there is any problem, it will become immediately apparent."

"I'm confused," I say. "Why do you want me to wait three months?"

"I want you to use this three month period to train your body to respond to the immunotherapy in the most effective way possible. I will speak to Dr. Chang and ask him to send me a copy of his protocol, from the very first step to the last. After I receive it, we will go through the protocol together and I will help you understand everything that will be occurring on a cellular level. Then, working together, we will create an audio tape that guides you step by step through the complete procedure. Your input will be crucial, for you will be the sole creator of the images you will use.

The tape will be approximately forty five minutes in length. Every day, for the next few months, you will work with the tape. Regular use of the tape will greatly assist in training your body to be in optimal working condition for receiving the actual immunotherapy treatments," James concludes.

"It's like training for a marathon," I say, excitedly.

"Exactly," James replies.

"I can do that," I say, feeling my optimism and fighting spirit beginning to return.

Armed with a growing conviction that I will be able triumph over the cancer, I am much more matter of fact when I inform family and friends of the recurrence. Responding to my strengthened conviction, they also are able to view this as an undesirable turn of events, that surely I will overcome. Not that there aren't tears, feelings of sadness, and deep pain around my unwelcome news. There certainly is. Both for myself and for others. But my natural optimism and fighting spirit helps to soften the blow, and my positive attitude is frequently contagious. I tell everyone I share the news with, that immunotherapy is the most promising new treatment for kidney cancer, and emphasize that I expect it to work. I tell very few people how slim the odds of a complete response are. In truth, I put that as far out of my mind as possible, and focus all my energies on a total and permanent triumph over cancer. It is effective the majority of the time, but there are also isolated periods when I am filled with fear. Actually, consumed by it. During one such episode, I sit at my computer and write the following piece which I title:

Memories

I am three years old, and I hide in the back of the hall closet, while mommy and daddy are fighting. Their voices are loud, and their words sound angry. I am very scared, and I suck on my blankey. The closet is a safe place to be. It is big, and it is soft, for I have pulled clothes onto the floor, and made a mattress to lie on. Nobody knows I am in the closet, so they cannot find me. After awhile, a door slams, and I know daddy has gone away again. I don't feel so afraid now, and I come out of the closet to look for mommy. She is crying, but when she sees me, she wipes her tears away, and hugs me very tight. Mommy tells me that everything is okay now. I want to believe her, but I am still afraid that daddy will come back and do bad things. I don't tell that to mommy. I pretend that I believe her.

I am fifty one years old, and I am afraid. I am looking for a safe place to hide, but I can't find one. Wherever I go, my fear goes with me. I have cancer, and I am afraid I am going to die. Much of the time, I don't feel afraid, because I believe I will heal from the cancer, and at those times I don't need a safe place to hide. When I feel filled with faith and trust, I love life, and want to immerse myself in it. When I feel afraid, the joys of life are too bittersweet, and I need to retreat. All the people who love me want me to live. They tell me that everything will be okay. I want to believe them, but when I'm afraid I believe the cancer has come back to do bad things, and that nothing will stop it. I don't tell that to the people who love me very often. It makes them very sad when I do. Instead, I pretend I believe them, and look for a safe place to hide until the fear goes away.

Reconnecting with God once again, I recognize how my feelings of abandonment and betrayal have completely isolated and separated me from knowing God's love. Letting my thoughts carry me back to God becomes one of the most meaningful parts of my journey toward healing. Once more, I feel my renewed partnership with God comfort and offer me hope, as I navigate toward a healing of body, mind, and spirit. I develop an unshakable belief that immunotherapy is a necessary step in my journey toward healing, and that through God's Infinite Wisdom, I am being given the opportunity to receive it. No longer do I feel lost or separated from God, for I know I am cherished and unconditionally loved. I may know what I want, but God knows what I need for my soul's growth. In accepting this as truth, I know peace once again. Not that I don't experience fear, for at moments I am still confronted by overwhelming terror. Still, my belief in my healing grows stronger every day, in direct proportion to the faith and trust I place in God, and for this I rejoice.

I can hardly believe what I have done this evening. While talking with God, I affirm once again how strongly I want to live, but that I will accept whatever decision God makes. I surrender to a Will much greater than my own, and offer it up to God. It is not easy to do, but I feel better for having done it. Talk about a letting go!

In my dream state I meet one of my inner guides. He says his name is Dr. Zydco, and he comes from India. He dresses in long, flowing, white robes, wears a white turban and jute sandals. His dark piercing eyes and serene smiling face radiates love and compassion. He wants me to open to the truth, so that I will prosper and live. He speaks with me about diet, imagery, and mantra meditation, but is especially emphatic about mantra meditation. He also shows me in great detail, the past eighteen months of my life prior to the onset of cancer.

"It is important for you to gain an understanding as to why this time frame is so relevant," he intones, and shares the following information with me.

Ongoing research shows that there appears to be a correlation between the onset of cancer and significant life changes that occur six to eighteen months prior to the onset. These changes are predominantly those that deal with major losses, such as the death of a loved one, divorce, undesired changes in significant relationships, both professional and personal, incapacitating accidents, and other major traumas. The theory is that these losses can depress and weaken the immune system, leaving ones body less able to defend itself against opportunistic invaders, such as cancer cells. Though many people are unaware of it, even a healthy body has some abnormal or cancerous cells. A strong and healthy immune system is able to destroy these cells quickly and efficiently, whereas a weakened immune system may be unable to effectively destroy all of them, allowing the cancerous cells to gain a foothold, multiply, and grow.

In retrospect, during this crucial eighteen month period, Brent and Tracy both leave for college, and my focus on parenting undergoes a radical change. I am excited to have the house to myself for the first time in my life. There is more time for me, but what do I want to do with it? Suddenly, there are many empty hours in my life. Will I find something new to fill them with? The loss of the old and familiar saddens me, while the visions of the new and unknown both excites and frightens me.

My work is satisfying, but it is not enough. Tapestry Counseling Center undergoes a major transformation as June moves to California and Pat accepts a full time position with another agency. Pat now sees clients at Tapestry Saturday mornings and two evenings a week, which means I basically work alone. Fifteen years of constant, supportive friendship and companionship, as well as a professional business partnership, is dramatically revised. Pat, June, and I have often stated that in many ways our relationship is like a marriage. Now that marriage has been radically altered, and I do not find it to my liking. Working alone much of the time, I experience a strong sense of loss. My involvement with Creating Results, though opening new doors to exciting work possibilities, cannot come close to replacing what I have just lost.

I am turning fifty, facing a mid-life shift, and also somewhat of a mid-life crisis due to my day to day world turning upside down. I am freer than ever to do whatever I want, but I am uncertain what that is. Life often feels scary to me, something akin to being in limbo, and I am uncomfortable being in limbo. I know change is inevitable, having gone through many previous changes in my life. I even know that limbo is part of the transition from the old to the new. But knowing something intellectually is nothing like feeling it emotionally.

Stan is a major plus, entering my life during a time both my parenting and partnership relationships are radically changing form. He represents all I have ever wanted in a relationship with a man. Some of the recent empty spaces in my life have been transformed through my relationship with Stan. Others dissolve as my own internal growth process accelerates. Still others disappear as I discover new and enjoyable pursuits. I find myself becoming more and more, the woman I want to be.

Based on the emphasis Dr. Zydco places on it, I decide to learn mantra meditation as soon as possible, and place the call that will change my life to Catherine "Chetana" Florida. Chetana is the founder of the Lighthouse Center, a non-profit organization dedicated to spiritual development through mantra meditation, chanting, and prayer. In addition, the center offers classes in Beginning and Advanced Meditation, Reiki, Astrology, Vegetarian Indian Cooking, Weekend Workshops, Children's Spirituality Classes, and Healing Night. Chetana is a gifted teacher of mantra meditation, an amazingly accurate psychic who offers channeled readings, a loving, compassionate Light worker, and a disciple of Gurudev Shree Chitrabanu, a Jain monk, philosopher, author, and a revered holy man of peace. She will also become my teacher and dearly beloved friend. I am indeed fortunate, for the next introductory mantra meditation class, will take place a week from now at Chetana's home. Despite her busy schedule, Chetana fits me in for a "reading" the day after the class, and I eagerly look forward to both.

"I think we should get married," Stan says that evening, very matter-of-factly.

"You what?" I say, not trusting my hearing.

"Get married," he repeats with a grin. "You and me. Married."

"Why now?" I ask, surprised at his timing. "Especially with my recurrence."

"I don't mean tomorrow," he laughs. "Sometime this summer. After you have completed your treatment. By then you will be cancer free."

"But why are you bringing it up now?" I persist, perplexed. "Why now, after this last bad news scan?"

Stan takes a deep breath, as he moves closer to me on the couch.

"I know I wanted to remarry," he says with complete candor, putting his arm around me, and drawing me to his side. "Ever since our talk around the campfire, I have known I wanted to marry you, but I have been cautious, because of your cancer. I didn't want to marry a woman who was dying, so I waited to see what the scans would show and bided my time. I told myself that when you had one year of clear scans I would ask you to marry me."

I interrupt. "Stan, I am more than confused. If that's how you feel, talking about marriage now just doesn't make sense."

"Let me finish," Stan says lovingly, and I fall silent.

"I was devastated just like you were, when you had the recurrence," he continues. "But then something miraculous happened. I saw how quickly you bounced back, how totally you refocused your energies on healing. I am impressed and in awe of such inner strength and power, and I know that I want to be joined to you and that incredible energy. Even if you were to die from this disease, which I believe with all my heart will not be the case, I would want to be with you every remaining day of your life. I am in love with an amazing woman. You inspire me, and I want to build a life with you."

I burst into tears, and bury my head against Stan's chest, hearing the steady, rhythmic beat of his heart. Stan tenderly lifts my head, and looks deeply into my eyes.

"Is that a yes?" he asks smiling at me.

"Yes," I smile back through my tears. "Yes Stan, I will gladly marry you, and I vow to be free of cancer when I do."

As we joyously embrace, a vision I had earlier this year of Stan and myself, radiant, in perfect health, and surrounded by family and friends on our wedding day, briefly flashes across my mind. Now this vision is preparing to manifest, so that our wedding day will be a celebration of love and of life.

A YEAR OF MIRACLES

CHAPTER 16

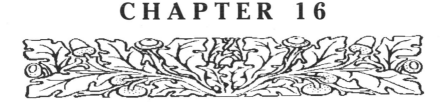

I Choose Life

I have increased my acupuncture sessions to twice a week in preparation for immunotherapy, as I believe acupuncture will strengthen my immune system, assisting it in working more effectively. Leaving my session with Charles and driving to a favorite restaurant, I look forward to my lunch date with Jennifer, who will be meeting me there. This is the first time we will spend a few hours alone since she learned of my recurrence. After embracing in greeting, I notice Jennifer looks sad, and lost in thought. Over salad and pasta, I learn why.

"I think maybe it's my fault that you developed cancer, and then had a recurrence," Jennifer says in a low voice, lips trembling.

"You had nothing to do with it," I say emphatically, dismayed at what I am hearing. "It's not your fault."

"Maybe I'm just bad luck for the people I love," she continues shakily. "First, my mother got cancer and died, and now you."

"Jennifer," I say gently, my heart breaking for the pain she's in, "love helps people heal. It doesn't make them sick, and it doesn't kill them. Your love makes me fight that much harder to live."

Jennifer raises a tear stained face, takes a deep breath and haltingly speaks. "But my mother died even though I loved her, and maybe you will also."

"I may die from cancer," I acknowledge, "although I believe I will live. Either way, your love is a gift to me, and I treasure it, just as your mother did. Your mother died knowing you loved her, which enriched and brightened her life."

Jennifer looks at me, a tremulous smile inching its way across her face.

I reach across the table, and stroke her hand.

"Just as your love enriches and brightens my life," I smilingly say.

Twenty of us are seated in Chetana's living room, waiting for the evening to begin. Most are new to meditation. Others, like myself, are meditators, but practice a different kind of meditation. A few long time mantra meditators and members of the Lighthouse Center have come to add their energies to our group. Chetana is a dynamic speaker. It is immediately apparent how strongly she believes in the benefits of mantra meditation. She talks about the profound changes in her life since becoming a meditator. They are impressive and inspiring.

Chetana tells us, "The mantra you will learn and meditate to is a powerful mantra of unconditional love, which connects you immediately with the God energy. Mantra meditation is really a cleansing of the nervous system. When you meditate regularly, anything that doesn't support Love, Light, and Order can't remain. Love and Light will make negative blockages dissolve in the physical, mental, and emotional bodies."

There isn't a sound in the room, and twenty pairs of eyes are riveted to Chetana's face.

"Love," Chetana simply states, "is the greatest healer of all."

After learning the mantra from Chetana, lights are dimmed, and we meditate to the mantra for twenty five minutes. I am at one with the mantra, and time passes quickly. It feels natural and effortless to meditate this way. Afterwards, Chetana asks us about our experiences meditating. As we circle the room sharing, I become aware that the group members feel like friends by now. I idly wonder if this is an added benefit of group meditation.

Chetana urges us to meditate twice a day for optimal benefits.

"Once a day," she states, "will be effective in greatly reducing your present stress level. Twice a day eventually will remove accumulated stresses from your past that are housed and stored in your body."

I make a silent commitment to meditate every morning and evening. Except for an occasional lapse, this is a practice I follow and expect to continue the rest of my life.

My reading with Chetana the following morning, is informative and enlightening.

Chetana snips off a small piece of my hair, and after asking for and receiving my permission to enter my vibrational field, holds the hair to her forehead. She remains silent a few minutes, while making contact with her guides.

"This is the last time the cancer energy will come up through your nervous system in this lifetime," she begins. "What I am telling you is a direct message from Spirit, who wants you to know that you will be permanently healed."

I feel tears of joy welling up behind my eyelids.

"Spirit says, you have released ninety percent of the cancer energy, but there is still ten percent you are holding onto. When it is released, you will be finished with cancer."

"Does Spirit show how to do that?" I ask, hoping Spirit will reply.

Chetana closes her eyes, connects with her guides again, and listens intently for a few minutes before responding. "Spirit shows me that the most efficient way to release the negative energy in your body, is through healing your mind and emotions of the resentment of injustices done to you by a family member early in your life."

My father I think immediately.

"As a young child I was very resentful that my father rejected and abandoned me, and it negatively colored my later years," I explain to Chetana. "But I have already done so much work on this anger and resentment."

"If you hadn't you wouldn't be here now. You have moved much more energy through you than you are aware of having moved. Now you have reached the last remaining layer and it has risen to the surface, ready to move out of your nervous system," she says. "Spirit shows that you are ready for a new growth step. The two come together. You take the new growth step and move forward. The final layer lifts out of your nervous system, and you are healed and finished with cancer."

"Does Spirit show steps to take?" I ask.

"Yes," Chetana says and outlines a number of things Spirit says for me to do.

"Make sure to do mantra meditation morning and evening," she begins.

I nod my head in agreement.

"Spirit also says to work with the affirmation I can have a happy, healthy, productive life now. They show you didn't know that growing up, because the people around you didn't set that example," she continues.

I think about that. "My mother loved me and believed in me," I say quietly, "but I didn't see from her life, or the lives of my relatives, that it was possible to have a happy, healthy, and productive life."

"And therefore, you didn't learn that program growing up," Chetana replies gently, nodding in agreement. "Spirit says that now is the time for you to live out this affirmation."

"I will," I promise.

"And to have Reiki healing."

"What is that?"

"It is a form of hands on healing, where the God energy comes through the hands of the healer," she explains. "I can give you the names of some Reiki healers, if you would like to pursue it."

"I would," I answer intrigued. "Very much so."

"And to learn and begin singing the "Navakar Mantra." Your Reiki healer can teach it to you. The two of you can sing it during the treatments, and you can sing it during the day."

"What is the Navakar Mantra?" I ask curiously.

"It is a very powerful healing prayer calling upon the Enlightened Beings to help you overcome your inner enemies. In India, documentation has shown that regular singing and chanting of the Navakar Mantra assists in healing a variety of ailments."

"I will learn it, and sing it," I promise.

Chetana falls silent once again, listening to her guides. After a long pause she speaks.

"Spirit says you must completely release any remaining negative energy around your father," she continues. "You must separate the human self from the Divine Self. Ask the Divine Self to send blessings, love, light, and forgiveness to your father. Sending the blessings, love, light, and forgiveness creates a boomerang effect. They arch back and heal the human self."

"I'll do that," I say. "Many, many times. I want to be completed with him."

"Cancer is an issue of anger from the past," she states in a clear and powerful voice. "As it surfaces in the physical body, the mental and emotional program will also come to the surface. Things that haven't been released from the nervous system. When you work with it now, send it love, light, and order as well."

I nod in agreement.

"Spirit says to have patience, faith, and trust," Chetana concludes. "Spirit shows me that you will heal."

I return home to find a large package outside the front door from Kal and Karen. Eager to find out what they have sent, I immediately tear open the box, and lift out a strange looking, but totally lovable being. He stands about a foot tall, and has a day-glow yellow oversized head and hands made of soft, pliable rubber. He sports a Jimmy Durante nose, and his smile, spreading from cheek to cheek, makes me respond with one of my own. His eyes are the deepest of blues, and house two white stars that swim in the black pupils of each eye. Outrageously oversized black rubber shoes, tied with thick white laces, add an additional comic touch. Over a soft black cloth body, he wears a bright yellow belted sweatshirt, and pinned to the top of his shirt is a large orange button that proclaims, "I BELIEVE IN YOU!!" Both the "I"s and exclamation marks are dotted in stars. Completing his persona, on the lower half of his sweatshirt is printed in bold, black, impossible to ignore double lettering:

FROYD
For Reality Of Your Dreams

A YEAR OF MIRACLES

Accompanying him, is a note from Kal and Karen. "Since we can't be with you every day, we send FROYD to keep you company. His message to you is our message to you. We believe in you, and know your dream of a complete healing will soon become a reality."

Grateful for the double affirmation of today, I hug FROYD and carry him into my room, placing him where I can be reminded of his message during the weeks and months that lie ahead.

With Thanksgiving only a few days away, my thoughts turn to a ritual I do every Thanksgiving. Sitting at my desk, I write my 1991 Thanksgiving list:

What I Am Thankful For

I am thankful for:
Stan being in my life, and our upcoming marriage.
My birth children, Sharon, Elyssa, and Brent.
My soon to be step children, Ari and Natalie.
My heart children, Tracy, Jennifer, and Adie.
The new, strong connection with Kal, Karen, Kris and Kirk.
Susan, Marilyn, Pat, June, Rose, Gwen, and many other loving friends.
My son-in-law Chuck, and Elyssa's partner Jeff, loving men who nurture my daughters.
Being Alive.
My increased appreciation of Life.
The lessons I am learning from cancer.
The work I do.
Having a love filled heart.
Being so loved by so many.
My health, despite the fact I have cancer.
Having my basic needs met.
My partnership with God
My expanding faith and trust.
My courage, strength, and ability to live life fully most of the time.
My creativity.

Meditation as a daily practice.
Immunotherapy.
James and Dr. Chang.
This computer and printer.
The lessons I am learning, even when I don't like
*   the form they take.*
Chetana Florida and the Lighthouse Center.
My sense of humor, even in times of sadness and
*   pain.*
Being Alive.
My mind.
My Celica.
My clients, who are teachers for me.
Having lived for 51 years.
Feeling such joy in feeling so fully alive.
Mocha, Shanti, Sue and Norm. [Brent's hamsters
*   who live at our house while he's at college]*
My essentially positive outlook on life.
Being Alive.

I read through the list I have just written, thankful to have so much to be thankful for.

Thanksgiving Day dawns bright and crisp. This year, for the first time, Tracy and I will be celebrating Thanksgiving at Stan's house. Stan's daughter Natalie will be preparing the holiday dinner, something she feels a strong desire to do. My children will be spending the day at their father's home. It has become a custom since our divorce to alternate holiday celebrations, and this one is his. Norm and his wife Carolyn, have graciously invited me for the holiday meal, and though I will drop by for dessert, I choose to spend the day with Tracy, Stan, Ari, Natalie, and some of their friends. I feel some discomfort around this decision, as this occasion is the first Natalie and I will be spending any significant amount of time together. With the subsequent passage of time, our relationship will deepen into a mutually warm, supportive, and loving one, but for now it is far from that. We are cordial to one another, but keep our distance. I respect Natalie's need to go slowly, and can understand why she does not welcome a new woman into her father's life. Natalie, in turn, respects me for understanding, and not trying to push her beyond where she is presently ready and able to go.

Ari is another story, altogether. There is no ambivalence or discomfort being with Ari. He has been Brent's best friend since first grade, has spent countless days and nights in our house, and frequently vacations with our family. Over the years, I have watched Brent and Ari grow to manhood. I have cheered them on, loved them, and comforted them when necessary. Ari has visited me at the hospital. He calls me from college to let me know he is rooting for me. Just recently, he and I have had a talk about my relationship with his dad.

Ari is direct. "It's strange to see my dad with someone other than my mom, but if my dad is going to be with anyone, I want it to be you. You make my dad happy, and he deserves to be happy. Besides," he adds hugging me, "I know you and I love you."

Ari is easy to be with. Always has been. Ari is family.

I am downtown, shopping for a birthday present at Falling Water, when I bump into Kay, whom I have not seen since just prior to my recurrence. I have not attended the past two writing classes, but plan on returning later this week. Kay seems visibly upset as we exchange greetings, and before I can update her, she begins to speak.

"I hear your cancer has returned, and I have a request to make of you," she says in a hushed voice. "I would like permission to put your name into a healing circle which will be meeting tonight. Twenty women will be in attendance, and the energies generated are very powerful and healing."

"You have my permission," I say, "for I appreciate all healing energies directed toward me, but how did you learn about the recurrence?"

"Carol came into the store last week, and told me."

I think back and remember Carol walking into the restaurant where Stan and I are dining. Carol is only a casual acquaintance of mine, but she and her husband know Stan through Chabad House, and he invites her to join us. During the meal we discuss my recurrence, and Carol voices compassion. But there is something underlying her concern that I can't put my finger on, and it leaves me feeling distinctly uncomfortable. I now realize Carol has gone across the street as soon as we part company, and informed Kay. I snap out of my reverie, and look at Kay.

"Strange as it may sound Kay, most of the time I am not that worried. I expect to heal," I say with conviction.

Kay smiles. "I have the sense you'll be around for a good long time."

"Me too," I agree laughing. "I'll probably end up being your oldest writing student. A genuine relic. A one of a kind antique."

It isn't until I leave the store that I feel my anger towards Carol build, and it continues escalating during the short drive home. I call Stan as soon as I walk into the house.

"She has no right to do that," I say angrily. "It's my business. It's up to me to tell who I want, when I want. I don't want people to pity me, or feel sorry for me."

"That isn't how people would necessarily feel," Stan suggests. "Did Kay feel that way?"

"No, she didn't. I know my friends and family don't, but I suspect Carol does. I also think she likes to spread bad news. It makes her feel important. And it makes me mad."

"I think something got triggered in you," Stan says gently. "Your response is much more intense than the situation warrants. And Carol may have told Kay, feeling she would be able to help you."

"I know," I agree wearily. "Carol represents something from my past that is working itself out of my nervous system emotionally. She is both a catalyst and a teacher for me, a reminder of something I need to acknowledge and release. Just don't tell me to be grateful to her yet. I probably will be later."

Stan laughs.

"I'm going to meditate now, and see what surfaces," I say testily. "Somehow, I suspect, that this is just the tail of the tiger."

A YEAR OF MIRACLES

Deep in meditation, I come face to face with the tiger. It is the same tiger about whom, in the winter of 1986, I write the following :

> *This ancient dream*
> *I sometimes glimpse*
> *is guarded by a tiger*
> *who will not yield,*
> *until I dance*
> *the dream awake.*

As a child, my mother is the only divorced adult I know. This is a source of resentment, shame, and sorrow for me, and I imagine for my mother as well, although neither of us ever acknowledges it. Unacknowledged, it remains unspoken between us, yet as real as the air we breathe, playing an essential part in our lives.

I am constantly teased and made fun of by merciless children, but much worse is my knowledge that neighbors pity us, and gossip behind our backs. I believe if I were good enough, my father wouldn't have abandoned me. Certain that all the adults know this as well, I keep my head bowed, eyes focused on the ground. That way I can avoid looks of pity, and knowing eyes that signal I am to blame.

Momma begs me over and over to hold my head up high. She insists I am as good as anyone else, but how can a daughter believe a mother who also isn't good enough? In desperation, momma sends me to a psychiatrist, but I don't utter a word. Even when some pervert sticks his hand into my panties, as I climb the steps to my appointment, I tell no one until I return home. I am convinced I am being punished because I am crazy and responsible for my father's leaving. Why else would momma want me to talk to a stranger?

I resent being different. I want to be like everyone else. I resent having rich distant relatives who help support us. I feel like a charity case. Shame, sorrow, pity, and not good enough are my constant childhood companions. Sticking closely to my side, they follow me wherever I go. Upon entering high school, thanks in large measure to momma's ongoing belief in me, I consciously choose to banish them, and replace them with new companions. They are named confidence, courage, self esteem, and popularity, and they serve me well.

With the recurrence of cancer, these hauntingly painful childhood companions resurface once more. I feel shame for having cancer, and fear that others will pity me. I feel not good enough. If I were, I wouldn't have cancer again. A deep river of sorrow flows through me whenever I consider the possibility of cancer ending my life. Especially now, with everything to live for.

I sob throughout most of my meditation. Gut wrenching, heart breaking sobs, coming from a secret place, buried deep within my soul. A place which I am acknowledging only now. The hidden room I have tried so hard to forget. I search for, and find the key that unlocks the door I've slammed shut so many long years before. As I turn the key and enter the gloomy, cobwebbed room, my old childhood companions, shame, pity, not good enough, and sorrow rush eagerly to my side. I greet them compassionately, extending my arms in friendship, forgiveness, and love. We embrace as sunlight pierces the darkness. Breathing deeply, I gently let go.

Talking about the upcoming immunotherapy, I learn from James that Dr. Chang has agreed to the three month delay, and is cooperative and supportive of this joint endeavor. James is awaiting the protocol which Dr. Chang is sending. At our next session, we will begin preparations for the immunotherapy tape. I am very pleased with this news, and my mood, which is lighthearted and exuberant, becomes even more expansive.

"There's an exercise I would like you to do before our next session," James says, looking directly at me.

"Sure," I say unsuspectingly. "Just tell me what it is."

"I want you to think about and then write why it would be okay to die," he says calmly.

"You what?" I explode, sitting bolt upright, not believing what I am hearing.

James repeats his request in the same soft spoken voice.

"I don't want to do that." I am adamant in my response. "I won't do it!! Why are you asking me to?"

"For a number of reasons. It's a very powerful exercise, and if you do it, some important revelations will emerge. These revelations can actually help strengthen your life force."

I take a deep breath and slowly center myself. I trust James implicitly. If he's asking me to do this, I will, although at the moment I can't think of a single reason why it would be all right to die.

James waits patiently while I compose myself and then continues. "There's another reason as well. You said in our earlier conversation that a 'deep river of sorrow flows through you, whenever you think about dying.' I believe this exercise will help lessen that sorrow."

"You know I don't want to die, James. You know how strongly I feel about living," I say peevishly.

"There's no doubt in my mind about that," he replies quietly. This exercise is not 'why I want to die.' It is 'why it would be okay to die.' There is a world of difference between the two."

"All right," I say resignedly, watching as my lighthearted mood evaporates. "I'll do it, but I still don't like it."

James looks at me compassionately. "I'm well aware of that Susan, and I'm looking forward to hearing what you write," he says with a smile.

"Just get it over with," I say to myself on the drive home. "Write it, and get it out of the way."

I walk into the house, drop my coat on the couch, and head toward the study and my computer.

"I'm not going to think about it," I announce, petting Mocha as she follows me into the room. "I'm just going to let my stream of consciousness flow, and trust whatever emerges."

Mocha barks in agreement, wags her tail, and settles by my side as I begin to write:

Why It Would Be Okay To Die.

*I wouldn't feel bad about my mother's life and
death.*

I could stop trying so hard.

I could totally let go.

I wouldn't have to prove myself.

I could be totally at peace.

*I could have a closer relationship with God,
Goddess, All There Is.*

I could release all stresses.

I wouldn't have money concerns.

It would be an adventure.

*My children are grown and don't "need" me. They
would miss me terribly, but they would be
okay.*

*I would have experienced the love I have wanted
my whole life.*

Death is a part of life. It's inevitable.

*I wouldn't be into "having to do it right." Especially
in regard to healing from cancer. The pressure
would be gone.*

*I had a near death experience in 1975. It was a
most wondrous, peaceful, loving feeling. I
chose to come back for my children.
Otherwise, I would have gone on. There isn't
anyone or anything "I have to" be here for,
although there is much "I want to" be here
for.*

*I would get to experience something new, and find
out if it is what I think it is.*

*I would be reunited with people I love who have
died, unless they have reincarnated by the
time I die.*

I would let go of my judgments of myself.

*I would stop putting off things until tomorrow, and
stop putting myself down for doing it.*

*I wouldn't have to experience advanced old age,
and see all the people I love die.*

I wouldn't have to figure out if my purpose for being

here now is really my purpose, and if it isn't, what is my purpose? And what if I don't have one?

I could completely detach myself from all earthly concerns.

I would have lived my life with few regrets. What really matters to me, I already have been blessed with.

I could stop being a healer to others, which I believe is a big part of my purpose here, and let death be the final healing for me.

I could stop being responsible for God knows what.

For most of my life, I have been in touch with this deep longing that has no name, but which I believe is my desire "to go home to God." I could.

I could shed my body and fly free. How exhilarating!!!!!!!

I don't know how much the work I am doing nourishes me now. I know I am very good at it, and many people heal as a result of it, but I'm not sure I want to keep on doing it indefinitely. I have ideas about what I want to do, but financially, I can't afford to. Dying would resolve this.

I could just let go, period. Let go of all stresses. All doubts. All fears. All insecurities. All cares. All concerns. All buried psychological motivations that I have no awareness of. Just one big letting go of my shadow side. I could stop trying.

I COULD JUST LET GO!!!!!!!

James is right on both counts I think as I read and reread what has arisen from within the depths of my soul. These new spiritual illuminations can assist in strengthening my life force, as I resolve the issues they raise. And the deep river of sorrow around dying doesn't feel quite as deep, or as sorrowful, as I connect with the positive and transcendent aspect of death. I can see that dying will be a wonderful adventure to explore some very distant day. One that will carry me back home to God. But as for now, more than ever before, I CHOOSE LIFE.

A YEAR OF MIRACLES

CHAPTER 17

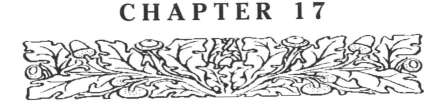

Healing From Within

This is my first time at the Lighthouse Center's Healing Night, and I am eagerly looking forward to it. Healing Night is open to adults and all children over the age of thirteen. There is no charge for Healing Night, and no one is turned away. Monetary contributions are accepted to further the work of the Lighthouse Center, but strictly on a voluntary basis. I know that many in need of healing have already been healed of a variety of physical imbalances. I look forward to adding my name to the list. Once the group gathers, Chetana explains to those of us new to Healing Night what will be occurring over the next few hours. First we will do a White Light Induction, followed by Mantra Meditation for twenty five minutes. This will enable us to become clearer channels for the Healing Energies, and assists us in opening to receive these Healing Energies. Those not familiar with Mantra Meditation are told to imagine a bright White Light emanating from within. They are to see this White Light totally surrounding them, and expanding to surround everyone gathered in the room.

"The healer is not doing the healing," Chetana emphasizes. "The healer is a channel for the Energies. The Healing Energy is coming from the God Source or Divine Conscious Mind. The healers also benefit from the Energy as it is channeled through their hands. Since the healer is channeling energy from an Unlimited Source, the healing is also Unlimited."

A YEAR OF MIRACLES

After meditation, the healing begins. Each healer pairs up with a healee. I find out that it is fine to talk, laugh, cry, or be silent. Whichever one desires. It is not necessary to concentrate or do anything special in order to channel or receive Healing Energies. That is the simple beauty of the healing process. Thereafter, about every ten minutes, the healers move on to work with a new healee. During the course of the evening, seven different healers will work with me.

It is during this first evening that I meet, and connect on a deep soul level, with a wonderful Reiki healer named "Bright Star," whom I will begin working with individually. Bright Star and I will meditate together, while she does Reiki healing on me. She will also pray with me and for me, teach me to sing and chant the Navakar Mantra along with other malas, and counsel and encourage me on my healing journey. This beautiful, gentle, gifted, loving woman will also become my friend.

Something is becoming clearer to me as the days go by. In my frantic exploration of alternative options, I am exhausting myself, raising my stress level, and driving myself crazy. I am discovering that by focusing so intently on healing from cancer, sometimes I tend to lose sight of the joys of daily living. At the same time, I am trying to let go, and let it be okay to heal into life or into death. This is the greatest challenge of all, for I do not feel at all neutral about the possibility of dying. Not even after having done "why it would be okay to die." More accepting? Yes. But neutral? Not at all. I am in love with life, and want many more years. Dying is not a part of my vision, though it has become more of a possibility in my current reality.

In the midst of a possible death sentence, I am creating the life I want. Stan and I will marry July 12th, and plan to build a new life together. I am focusing my life as if I will live to be a hundred, and doing what I would be doing if cancer weren't in my reality. I remember after George's two recurrences and a very uncertain future, how he and Sheila courageously went ahead and had a second child. Michael is now twenty one, and George is alive, active, healthy and cancer free. It takes courage to create life in the face of uncertainty, but unless I continue to do just that, I will become one of the living dead, and then it would really be okay to die. In fact it would be preferable.

I know my healing has to come from within. I know I need to get out of my own way and let the healing in. Somehow, I must find the way to create a balance, where I focus on living, accept that I may die sooner than I want, and live each day I have to its fullest. That means deciding on my own program, sorting out the myriad alternatives, choosing those that intuitively speak to me, and creating a way of life that I can live with, and if need be, die with as well. But as of now, my focus is on healing into life, and of that I couldn't be clearer.

It takes me another week to sort out all the available alternatives, and decide on the ones I instinctively feel will work for me. This is one of the most important steps I take on my path to healing, for it is necessary to both believe in, and be comfortable with the choices that I make. In addition to a low fat, high fiber, predominantly vegetarian diet, mega-vitamin and mineral supplements, exercise in the form of a daily half hour to hour walk with Mocha, acupuncture to strengthen my immune system, twice a week sessions with James, and Reiki healing with Bright Star, my days look like this:

Mornings I awaken by 7:00 a.m. and spend the next two and a half hours focusing on my healing program. Afterwards, I eat breakfast, shower, and start my day. During this intense healing phase, I continue to work part time and schedule my clients in the afternoon or early evening. My mornings begin like this:

> *Prayer and Giving Thanks to God. [15 minutes]*
> *Deep abdominal breathing to bring oxygen to my*
> *   internal organs. [10 minutes]*
> *Imagery to shut off the blood supply to the tumor.*
> *   [5 minutes]*

The Lazaris morning tape. [15 minutes]
Chanting the Navakar Mantra. [15 minutes]
Mantra Meditation. [25 minutes]
Preparation for Immunotherapy Tape. [40 minutes]
Stretching my body. [10 minutes]
Running on the Rebounder to exercise the Lymphatic System. [15 minutes]

Early to mid afternoon I set aside thirty minutes to do the following practices:

Chanting the Navakar Mantra. [15 minutes]
Imagery to shut off the blood supply to the tumor. [5 minutes]
Wolf visualization, where I see a pack of strong, hungry gray wolves devouring weak and frightened cancer cells, then patrolling the area on the lookout for any strays. [10 minutes.] The Wolf is my Spirit Animal, and I have taken Wolf as my middle name.

I set aside an hour or more every evening and do the following practices:

Imagery to shut off the blood supply to the tumor. [5 minutes]
Chanting the Navakar Mantra. [15 minutes]
Mantra Meditation. [25 minutes]
Running on the Rebounder. [15 minutes]
Prayer and Giving Thanks to God. [15 minutes]

I find both comfort and empowerment in the practices I have chosen. Although it requires strict discipline on my part to maintain them, my desire to heal is so overwhelmingly strong, that the discipline becomes effortless. Being so totally and completely focused on my healing makes it possible for me to do whatever it takes to realize my heartfelt desire. These practices, along with immunotherapy, and the ever-present love and support of God, family, and friends, will turn out to be a winning combination.

James explains how we will be working in partnership to create the audio tape which I will use during the actual immunotherapy. I will be birthing the visual images described on the tape. Together, we will be creating a taped script which we anticipate will enhance the effectiveness of the experimental immunotherapy protocol tenfold.

"It is very similar to Pavlovian conditioning," James says. "We will be pairing three conditioned stimuli, [CS] with three unconditioned immunizing stimuli. [UCIS] The conditioned stimuli will be multi-sensory."

"Please explain them again," I say. "This is more confusing to me than I like to admit. The truth is I never was very good in science."

James laughs. "We've already agreed on all three of them. You actually created the symbols and images. You just didn't realize they would be called conditioned stimuli."

"Again," I insist. "This still sounds like gibberish to me, and I need to understand it precisely."

"The first conditioned stimuli [CS] is the image of floating on your back in a cool pond, surrounded by a densely wooded area of cedar trees. You lie there peacefully, the tall cedar trees completely enveloping you. There is a small opening within the circle of trees that allows a cone of sunlight to filter through. The sunlight beams down on your thighs, and as you lie in the cool water, the scent of cedar permeates the air. You are mindful of your breath, and the rise and fall of your abdomen."

"I understand that one," I say excitedly. "That image is for the immunizing vaccination in my thighs. The one that combines my irradiated cancer cells and BCG, and that vaccination is considered the unconditioned immunizing stimuli. [UCIS] We will be pairing the two together."

James smiles and nods. "Using the tape, you will feel the energy of the sun enter your body, as you say silently to yourself, "Enter and Heal." You will visualize your immune system, located in your groin area, being stimulated. You will also visualize killer cells and other T cells being born, specifically designed to fight and destroy the tumor cells growing in you."

The second conditioned stimuli [CS] is a second cone of sunlight filtering through the trees, focusing at the base of your breastbone. This energy beam is what you have named Divine White Light, and it enters your body through the catheter which will be in place at the base of your breastbone. This Divine White Light will be paired with the potent lymphokine activated killer [LAK] cell infusion, which Dr. Chang will grow in the laboratory from the lymph nodes he will remove from your groin. These LAK cells are the second unconditioned immunizing stimuli. [UCIS] On your tape you will visualize the LAK cells being composed of Divine White Light, coursing through your body in search of the weak, confused cancer cells, and successfully finding them."

"The third conditioned response [CS] will be an intensely energetic laser like form of the beam of Divine White Light, which flows into your catheter in intermittent pulses. This laser like beam will be paired with the Interleukin-2 [IL-2] infusions, which are the third unconditioned immunizing stimuli. [UCIS] During this portion of the tape, you will feel the IL-2 enter your body in the form of this pulsating Divine White Light, and you will say silently to yourself, "Stimulate and Heal." IL-2 is responsible for stimulating your LAK cells to produce their cancer fighting bullets. With the help of the tape you will visualize the LAK cells and IL-2 binding. You will see them producing more and more bullets, and shooting the bullets into the cancer cells. Then you will see the cancer cells leaking and bursting."

"I see butterflies shooting the bullets out of their antennae." I speak excitedly as I clearly visualize them. "There are thousands of beautiful brightly colored butterflies flying about. They are totally absorbed in creating an arsenal of cancer fighting bullets, and shooting them into the cancer cells that make up the tumor on my rib."

"Wonderful imagery," James responds enthusiastically, and continues.

"You will then visualize IL-2 stimulating special scavenger cells to produce a substance called Tumor Necrosis Factor, [TNF] which is lethal to cancer cells and quickly kills them. You will observe the TNF coating the cancer cells, and watch the cancer cells being destroyed."

I am excited once again. "Clouds. Huge rain filled clouds. They are stuffed so full that they have no choice but to open up. And the ensuing downpour saturates and drowns the cancer cells." I laugh in delight, and James laughs with me.

"You will also visualize other scavenger cells called macrophages entering the area. You will tell them to "clear the debris," and they will obey," James continues.

"Elephants," I shout, extremely pleased with myself. "Hungry elephants, using their trunks to clean up all the dead cancer cells."

"Good," James says. "I like all three of your images."

"Me too," I agree. "I see them so clearly. It will be fun working with them, and getting to know them better."

"There is one last part," James says smilingly. "After you have finished your healing session for the day, you will visualize yourself standing up in your pond, and walking over to the far corner, where there is a waterfall. You will stand under the waterfall, and let its cooling waters cleanse you of all toxic effects of this treatment. When you are ready, you will walk back into the woods, and as a final closing gesture of acceptance, you will send thoughts of loving kindness, thoughts of forgiveness, and compassionate thoughts to yourself."

"That is beautiful," I say. "The imagery is wonderful, and I am really looking forward to working with this tape. When will you have it ready for me?"

"Later this week," James replies.

"Thank you James," I say appreciatively, "but there is something else on my mind that I need your help with. I understand the conditioned and unconditioned stimuli [CS and UCIS] and the pairing of them. But I'm not sure how that pairing works. Would you explain it to me?"

"When you pair the conditioned and unconditioned stimuli, [CS and UCIS] a bi-directionality develops between your immune system and your central nervous system. Due to this bi-directionality, the specific immune responses which are produced by the immunizing vaccination, the LAK cells, and the IL-2, can be reactivated, focused, and enhanced through subsequent exposure to the conditioned stimuli." [CS]

"So the more I work with the tape which is programmed with the three conditioned stimuli [CS], the stronger my responses will become," I say, pleased to finally understand this scientific jargon.

"Exactly," James replies. "It is this reactivation and focusing of the specific immune responses which brings about both your enhanced resistance to tumor cell growth, and the regression of your tumor. This form of classical Pavlovian conditioning allows you to influence the inner workings of your body through repeated exposures to the three conditioned stimuli." [CS]

"I'll use the tape every day," I promise. "At least once a day. Maybe more."

"Excellent," James replies, sounding pleased.

"Just promise me one thing," I say barely suppressing the laughter that threatens to erupt.

"What is that?" James asks in all seriousness.

"Promise me, that a lasting side effect of Pavlovian conditioning won't be my uncontrolled salivating at the sight of Mocha's dog food."

I am unable to keep a straight face a moment longer, and peals of my laughter burst forth noisily, and fill the room.

"I think if you sent a letter to the Lubavitcher Rebbe, asking for his blessing, prayers and help in your healing, that it would be beneficial," Stan says thoughtfully.

"Why?" I ask. "What made you think of that?"

"I was talking with Rabbi Goldstein, and he actually suggested it," Stan answers. "I thought it was a good idea, so I'm passing it along. Especially after what Aahron told me."

"So tell me," I say, my curiosity aroused.

"Aahron says that the Rebbe, who is in his eighties, visits the grave of his father, the former Lubavitcher Rebbe, three times a week. There, he reads all the letters he receives for help, prays over them, blesses them, and leaves them on his father's grave." Stan pauses a moment. "Aahron says that many miracles occur for the people the Rebbe blesses and prays for. He says to let the Rebbe know where and when the immunotherapy will be taking place, and to leave the rest to the Rebbe."

"You met the Rebbe when you traveled with Aahron to the Lubavitcher community in Crown Heights shortly after Lynne died," I say reflectively.

"Yes I did, and he is a very holy man. I am awed by the Godliness he radiates." Stan smiles, remembrance lighting his face. "When the Rebbe greeted me, he said something very wonderful was about to occur in my life. Something that would bring great joy into my life again. Shortly after that, Ari invited me to your fiftieth birthday party, and the rest is history."

"I will write to the Rebbe today," I say thoughtfully. "I was already planning on writing the Crystal Cave."

"What is the Crystal Cave?" Stan asks.

"The Crystal Cave is comprised of a group of people who are closely connected with Lazarus. They help people who contact them, by sending them Healing Energy."

"By all means do it," Stan says supportively.

"And I had planned on calling Silent Unity, and asking them to pray for me. I will contact the Rebbe, the Crystal Cave, and Silent Unity today. As you know," I say stroking Stan's hand, "I welcome all miracles that come my way."

I fall silent for a moment, as the vision I had last March springs full blown into my consciousness. Once again I am surrounded, further than the eye can see, by a circle of people all sending healing energy to me.

"Stan," I say, barely able to contain my excitement, "there is something else I am going to do. I will send a letter to everyone I know, inviting them to be part of my Healing Circle. I will ask them to focus specific energies on me, during the time I will be receiving immunotherapy. I will share what I will be doing, and ask them to do the imagery with me. I believe that vision last March was a message from God, and I am going to act on it."

"What a wonderful idea," Stan says with an excitement that matches mine.

A YEAR OF MIRACLES

"I can hardly wait," I say throwing my arms around Stan. "Just imagine how incredibly powerful all that healing energy focused directly on me will be. I feel so strongly a miracle will occur, and I will be healed."

After Stan leaves I dial Silent Unity. The kindly, compassionate woman who answers and prays with me, reminds me they will pray for my healing continuously for the next thirty days. I only need to call or write every thirty days, and I will receive continual prayer for as long as I need it. Thanking her, I hang up the phone, feeling part of an extended community of loving, spiritual beings.

Seated at my computer, and keeping the momentum going, I write two letters. One to the Rebbe. One to the Crystal Cave. I decide to compose and send the letter to those people I would like to be part of my healing circle, closer to the actual date of my treatment. The letters I do write, are as follows:

Dear Rebbe,

I am a fifty one year old woman who loves God, and tries my best to do mitzvahs [good deeds] on a daily basis. This spring I was diagnosed with advanced kidney cancer, that had spread to my left hip, liver, and second and seventh ribs. I had surgery and radiation therapy, and was free of cancer for six months. In November, I learned the cancer had recurred in my seventh rib.

I am scheduled for immunotherapy in early February at the University of Michigan Hospital. It will be administered by Dr. Alfred Chang. I very much desire to live, and I am writing to ask for a blessing from you. Also, if there is anything you could suggest I do, so that God will be merciful and grant me life, I will joyfully do it. Thank you Rebbe.

Dear Crystal Cave,

This spring I was diagnosed with advanced kidney cancer, that had metastasized to my left hip, liver, and second and seventh ribs. I had surgery and radiation, and was scheduled for immunotherapy, which was postponed, because the cancer my doctor thought had spread to my liver disappeared. Truly a miracle. Since then I have worked with many Lazaris tapes, as well as having attended the Alchemy of Adversity seminar. I have looked at many of my beliefs, processed and changed them, and worked with my shadow side. I have strengthened my relationship with myself, my Higher Self, Future Self, and God, Goddess, All There Is... as well as the significant people in my life. I am doing all I know how to do.

In November, a CAT scan showed the start of a cancerous tumor on my seventh rib. This devastated me, because I believed the cancer was gone for good. It had not been visible on my CAT scans during the past six months. I am now scheduled for immunotherapy in early February, at The University of Michigan Hospital, which will be administered by Dr. Alfred Chang. Medically, this is the most powerful treatment available for advanced kidney cancer, so I am more than willing to go through it. I very much desire to live a long, healthy, happy, productive life. I will be getting married this July, and am making many exciting life changes. I feel strong, healthy, and very much alive. I am in love with life.

I am writing to ask for healing energy sent my way. In addition, if there is anything I am overlooking, or still need to clear out, please help me understand what needs to be done. And last, but certainly not least, if it is possible, I would appreciate receiving a consultation with Lazaris on the floating schedule. I thank you in advance, for the love, light, and healing, you will be sending my way.

I stuff the letters into envelopes, address, and stamp them. Unwilling to wait until tomorrow for the letters to be collected by the postman, I bundle up in my down parka, and on this snowy December 1st, arrive at the post office just in time for the last mail pick up of the day. Driving home, the freshness of falling snow transforming the familiar streets, I find beauty and hope in all that surrounds me.

The next few weeks fly by, with doubled holiday preparations, because I celebrate both Chanukah and Christmas. Growing up in my Orthodox Jewish household, our family always celebrates Chanukah, the Festival of Lights. It is a holiday a child's dreams are made of. Brightly wrapped presents for eight consecutive nights. Momma's delicious potato latkes. Singing Chanukah songs. Chocolate candy coins wrapped in gold foil, that taste as rich as they look. Playing dreidel with a handful of pennies. Happy when I win, but not unhappy if I lose. And every night for eight nights, lighting the ornate Chanukah Menorah, just like everyone else I know. Walking to the synagogue in the evening with momma and Kal, it appears as if every household in our neighborhood has a lit menorah in the window, illuminating the darkened streets and lighting our way.

To see a Christmas tree is a rare sight indeed, and it is not until I grow older, make some Christian friends, and move beyond the confines of my immediate neighborhood, that I am introduced to Christmas. I love the holiday of Christmas, the smell of cookies baking in the oven, the story of Rudolph the Red Nosed Reindeer, leaving milk and cookies for Santa Claus, the festivities, and the gaily wrapped presents lying under a beautifully decorated, brightly lit Christmas tree. Although I am uncomfortable with the religious aspect of the holiday due to my strong Jewish upbringing, I am somehow able to separate that part from the rest, and enjoy Christmas from a perspective I feel comfortable with.

Now, in years when both holidays occur simultaneously, it is not unusual to see a Chanukah menorah and a Christmas tree in my living room, and presents gaily wrapped in Chanukah and Christmas paper nestled side by side. As I see it, both Chanukah and Christmas celebrate Light, Miracles, and God's Love for All People. A time of Peace on Earth. Goodwill to All, regardless of race, religion, or creed.

Stan and I are at Chabad House, where for the first time, I assist as he make his famous potato latkes, [pancakes] which will feed the hundred congregants who gather to celebrate Chanukah. Aahron and Esther are warm, welcoming, and accepting of my spiritual path, though it is different from theirs. They make me feel at home, and part of their family, the congregation, and the larger Jewish community. As the lights on the menorah burn brightly, commemorating the miracle of one day's worth of oil keeping the lamps in the ancient temple burning for eight full days, I bow my head in prayer, and give thanks to God for the modern day miracle I believe is about to unfold.

I am at Stan's house several nights later, where once again he prepares his famous potato latkes for the thirty five people who have gathered to celebrate Chanukah. We eat the hot, tasty latkes with applesauce and sour cream, and play dreidel. Everyone invited receives a Chanukah present. Stan tells the story of Chanukah, and lights the intricate menorah. We sing songs and gather to talk in small groups. Although it is bitter cold outside, the warmth that radiates through the house makes it feel like a summer day.

Natalie's friend Andy has come to Michigan to spend Chanukah with her. He is 22, tall and lanky, wears a baseball cap and sports an infectious grin. The cap hides a head made prematurely bald from the side effects of chemotherapy. Andy has been battling cancer for three years. It has slowed him down, and tired him out, but it has not removed the grin from his face, or the optimism from his heart. I am touched by his beauty, and say a silent prayer for his full recovery. The world can use more Andys. We sit opposite one another when the latkes are served. Andy doesn't have much of an appetite, and eats very little. Yet he sparkles. He laughs. He engages people in conversation. He doesn't appear to feel sorry for himself. Andy has great presence for one so young. He emanates courage, dignity, and strength. No one at the Chanukah celebration knows it yet, but whereas I will live, Andy will not. His death, just a couple of years later, will come as a great blow to Natalie. I too will shed tears for the loss of such a beautiful spirit, but give thanks that I had the opportunity to meet him, even if it was for the briefest of times.

It is Christmas Day, and our family is gathering for brunch and the exchange of presents. Sharon and Chuck enter, cheeks red from the cold, arms loaded with presents, followed by Elyssa and Jeff, Jennifer and Jon. Brent, Ari, and Tracy, just barely awake, leave the warmth of their beds and pad barefoot into the kitchen. Stan and I hand out steaming mugs of coffee and hot chocolate as a tantalizing aroma from the quiches baking in the oven permeates the air. As the crackling fire dances in the fireplace, adding its own delightful fragrance, I look around at the faces of those so dear to me, and am transported in time to the previous Christmas.

Unlike me, Stan does not celebrate Christmas. Chanukah is the holiday he, Lynne, Natalie, and Ari have always observed. Because Ari is Brent's best friend, he is allowed to spend Christmas with our family, but this exception is granted only because of the closeness between the two boys. Natalie has felt jealous every Christmas that Ari has spent at our house, but I will not learn this until after we have formed a close and loving bond. Once Stan and I marry, Natalie will begin celebrating Christmas with the rest of the family, perhaps with the greatest joy and enthusiasm of us all.

Stan is in a quandary when I invite him for Christmas Day brunch. He definitely would enjoy being with us, but there is a problem. The thought of celebrating Christmas causes Stan considerable discomfort. Though he knows we do not celebrate the religious aspects of the holiday, he still feels uneasy. I make certain Stan knows I understand his feelings, and will respect his decision. If he feels uncomfortable, I would rather he not be there. We agree to leave it open ended. Either way is fine with me. The decision rests solely with Stan.

Christmas morning everyone gathers. No Stan in sight.

"I guess he decided not to come," I say to Marilyn who has flown in for the holidays.

"It looks that way," she agrees.

Just then the doorbell rings.

"I'll get it," Marilyn says cheerily, throwing the door wide open.

I gasp in disbelief, as an animated elf singing Christmas Carols enters the house. He is dressed in green tights, rust colored boots that reach his knees, a blousey cream colored silk shirt, a gold and blue brocade vest, and a wide brown leather belt, with a large, striking bronze buckle. A green velvet three cornered cap perches jauntily on his head. It is a perfect foil for his pointy elf ears, and bright orange whiskers. Over his shoulder he carries a colorful knapsack, filled to overflowing with Christmas presents.

"I'm Elwood Elf," he announces in a loud booming voice. "Santa's helper. Bringing presents, for all good girls and boys."

"Welcome Elwood," I say, choked with laughter. "Put down your knapsack and stay awhile. You've come to the right house. Lots of good girls and boys are gathered here."

I am brought out of my reverie by the ringing of the buzzer, which signals the quiches are ready to come out of the oven. Eating brunch, surrounded by those I love, mindful and grateful for the blessing of loved ones, and savoring this moment of life, an unbidden thought flashes across my mind.

"Maybe, this will be your last Christmas," it tauntingly whispers. "You had better make the most of it."

There is a bittersweet fragrance in the air that only I can detect. And it didn't exist just a moment ago.

A YEAR OF MIRACLES

It is New Year's Eve, and Stan and I are in Chicago. Having splurged, we are checked into a suite at a luxurious hotel, well known for its excellent restaurant and gourmet chef. I have bought a new purple dress for the occasion, and feel feminine and attractive. Stan looks handsome in his suit, tie, and dress shirt, attire he seldom wears. Seated for dinner, our window seat allows us a view of the brightly lit Chicago skyline. There is a bottle of champagne on our table and we are toasting the New Year.

"To 1992, and our wedding day," I say, feeling sentimental.

We touch glasses and drink.

"To 1992, and your complete healing," Stan says with a smile.

Once again we touch glasses and drink.

"To our love, forever and a day," we simultaneously say. Laughing delightedly, we link arms and sip the champagne.

We toast to God. To life. To miracles. To our children. Our family. Our friends. James and Dr. Chang. For two people who seldom drink, a bottle of champagne goes a long way.

We celebrate the New Year our favorite way, wrapped in one another's arms, giving and receiving mutual pleasure. The passion between us is explosive. There is nowhere either of us would rather be. I fall asleep, satiated, content, and overjoyed that 1992 has arrived. I am more than ready to take my leave of 1991.

During the night, I dream that there is a huge, dumb, deformed giant on the loose, whose goal is to kill all the people he can. He frequently succeeds, because he is so frightening to people, that the very sight of him terrifies them. This intense terror paralyzes his victims. Unable to defend against him, they are easily disposed of. One day the giant comes for me, and we engage in a life or death dance. The giant looks for any opportunity to kill me, but I disentangle myself from his grip before he can succeed. My strategy is in refusing to become so terrified of him that I cannot fight. I save myself by not succumbing to my fear. This allows me to think clearly, and do what is necessary to outwit the giant and live.

The dream jolts me awake, and I record it on the first page of my new gray wolf journal. I know without a doubt that the giant is cancer. Though my cancer is small in size, it looms large in my life, for I know it is capable of killing me. The dream clearly states, that as long as I don't let fear immobilize me, I can emerge victorious and live. Grateful to receive this message, and vowing to live by it, I silently give thanks.

As I am falling asleep, somewhere in that mystical space between awake and asleep, an important message is revealed to me.

"If I create my own destiny, it will be a wonderful one, but if I allow others to determine my destiny, it will not be to my liking."

That both the dream and the message come at the very start of the New Year, I take as a powerful sign that I will heal into wholeness.

While Stan is showering, I place the Runes, the Angel Cards, and the Medicine Cards on the table in the sitting room. I focus and center myself, connect with the love of God, and ask for an overview of 1992. Reaching into the bag, I draw the Rune of Harvest, One Year, Fertile Season.

The message is that the harvest, the deliverance, will occur this year. I have prepared the ground, planted the seeds, and am cultivating with care. I need to continue to persevere. Although the outcome is in the keeping of God's Will, it is very likely that I will succeed. I recall drawing this Rune in the hospital last March. One full year has almost passed. I believe this year will be the one in which I will harvest what I have sown, both in my healing from cancer, and in my marriage to Stan. Things are coming full cycle, and the time of harvest is almost within sight.

The Angel Card of Healing I draw harmonizes with the Rune of Harvest, as does Deer, whom I draw from the Medicine Cards. Deer represents the quality of gentleness, and is a reminder to use gentleness of spirit in healing of all kinds. By applying gentleness I will connect with Sacred Mountain, my centering place of serenity, and Great Spirit will guide me along the path of healing. I joyously write the messages for 1992 in my journal. When Stan emerges from the shower, I am eager to share the messages with him.

We spend much of the next day window shopping on Michigan Avenue. Walking in and out of stores. Trying on lots but buying little. Kissing in doorways. Huddling together. Seeking shelter from the cold wind. Laughing as three teenagers in a horse drawn carriage shout "nice wig lady," on seeing my windswept hair. Windy City is a fitting name for Chicago, especially along Lakeshore Drive, but I really don't mind. As that famous old song says, "I've got my love to keep me warm."

That evening we spontaneously buy tickets for a play entitled, "Prelude To A Kiss." We know nothing about the play, but the title appeals to us, and we decide to see it. As we exit the theater and duck into a restaurant for a late night snack, Stan turns to me.

"The play makes me think of our relationship," Stan says grinning.

"How do you mean,?" I ask, warming my hands on a hot mug of coffee.

"There is a marriage taking place, and there also is a life threatening illness that gets turned around," he answers. "And although the dynamics are different than ours, the couple gets to live happily ever after."

"Like us," I say quietly.

"Exactly," Stan responds. "I view seeing this play as a sign, that at the time of our wedding, you will be completely free of cancer."

We raise our mugs, bring them together, and drink.

Upon returning to the hotel, Stan places a yizkor [memorial] candle for Lynne on the coffee table in our sitting room. According to the Hebrew calendar, tonight marks the second anniversary of Lynne's death. In Judaism, this is observed by saying special prayers for the dead, and lighting a memorial candle, which burns for twenty four hours. I watch Stan recite the mourners kaddish and other prayers. I see him reverently light the candle, and watch as the flame dances higher. Lynne's soul is ascending another level, I think, and this thought makes me happy.

The next morning I awaken before Stan, slip out of bed, and walk into the sitting room to meditate. The yizkor candle burns brightly, and I sit opposite it. Prior to meditating, I invite Lynne's spirit to join me, if it wishes to. After entering a very deep state of meditation, I have a crystal clear image of Lynne. She is dressed in a long, white, shimmering robe. She appears youthful, vibrant, and radiant, the way she did before she became ill. Lynne gracefully glides towards me, and takes both my hands in hers. A powerful jolt of energy, much like an electric current, travels through my body.

"I have come to tell you something important," Lynne says, in a voice both soft and lyrical. "I have interceded with God, on your behalf and on Stan's. God has been merciful. You will be healed of cancer."

"Thank you Lynne," I say, overcome with a torrent of emotion. "May you always be blessed for your great love and compassion."

Lynne smiles a smile I can only describe as angelic, and is gone as suddenly as she appeared. I come out of meditation, immediately awaken Stan, and share what has just occurred.

Tears roll down Stan's cheeks as he hears me out. "That is Lynne's way," he says, in a voice choked with sentiment. "Her way is always to act from love."

A YEAR OF MIRACLES

CHAPTER 18

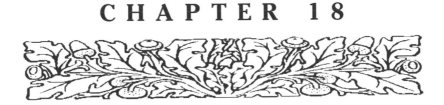

A Healing Circle

The thought of having a CAT scan the following morning is somewhat unnerving. This is the scan that will define and measure any new tumor growth during the past two months. My worst case scenario of cancer running rampant throughout my body, triggers the fear. I want the tumor:
>   a) to have miraculously disappeared, or if
>   that isn't possible,
>   b) to have remained the same size, or if that
>   is not the case,
>   c) to have grown only slightly.

Any other outcome is unacceptable.

Asking for help regarding my fear, I once again draw the Rune of Harvest. It encourages me to keep my spirits up, and trust in a beneficial outcome. As I reflect upon this Rune, an image of the dumb, deformed giant comes to mind. I take this as a sign that now is the time to remember, and act upon the message in my dream. As long as I refuse to allow my fear to terrorize me, I can emerge victorious.

That night I dream I am with Dr. Chang, who is the recipient of an award for the important cancer research he is conducting. I congratulate him, and acknowledge just how much he deserves this recognition. Dr. Chang smiles, and thanks me. Looking very pleased, he casually mentions that my latest scan shows the tumor to be quite small. Just hours later, I leave for the scan which goes without incident, and await the test results in a relaxed and trusting frame of mind.

A YEAR OF MIRACLES

Elaine, a friend and member of Gwen's group, whom I have asked to be a support person, calls that evening. Meditating during my scan, Elaine has received a message she wishes to share.

"The message," Elaine states lovingly, "is that there are additional lessons for you to learn around faith. When your faith is being challenged, that is when you need to hold on the tightest."

"That is when it becomes most difficult to do," I interject, "but I'm doing my very best."

"I know you are," she readily agrees, "and I admire you for it."

Thank you for your vote of confidence," I answer, feeling affirmed .

"I can still see the tumor on your rib, and it is approximately the same size," Elaine says gently.

"Your vision matches mine," I reply calmly. "I can sense the tumor is still inside me, with perhaps the slightest change in size. That is acceptable for now, for I stand strong in faith. Soon enough, the tumor will be gone for good."

Dr. Chang calls to say the tumor has barely grown these past two months. This means that the work I have been doing has altered the usual course of the tumor's progression. Normally the tumor would grow as much, or more, in this two month period as it did the previous two months. But its growth is significantly less. My body is being a very good friend to me. It is working hard to fight the cancer, and it is being successful.

"Thank you body," I say with gratitude. "I love you. Keep up the good work."

"I knew you could do it," James says when I relay the news. "I don't think you give yourself enough credit."

"For what?" I ask feeling confused.

"For just how powerful you are in influencing the course of your cancer," he responds with a smile.

"Maybe you are right," I agree, "but as my friend Scarlet says, I'll think about it tomorrow. All I want to do today is celebrate the good news."

170

My New Year's reading with Chetana is once again enlightening and life affirming. The Angels of Healing, Light, and Joy that I draw will be the primary angels watching over me throughout 1992.

"I drew the Angel of Healing on New Year's Day," I say happily.

"Spirit showed it to you then, and shows it to you now," Chetana responds. "You are doubly blessed."

"Double Healing Angels," I reply joyfully.

"To assist in healing from cancer," Chetana adds, eyes sparkling.

"What else does Spirit show?" I ask in a serious voice.

Chetana falls silent, listening to her guides. "Spirit shows me two previous lifetimes where you desperately wanted to die."

"Why?" I query, curious, but somehow not surprised.

"In one lifetime you were severely tortured in an attempt to make you betray others. All you would answer was, 'I want to die. Just let me die.' Finally, mercifully, you did die without betraying anyone," Chetana tenderly says.

"In the second lifetime you were sold into a life of servitude, into a marriage with a wicked man. You felt helpless, and hopeless, with no apparent way out. You spent that lifetime wanting to die."

Chetana pauses a few moments before continuing. "The root cause of this death wish is from those previous lifetimes, but the seed was carried into this lifetime through your nervous system. What you are doing now is clearly choosing life, thereby helping your body release and transform this desire to die. The programming you carried into this lifetime is not something you have a conscious awareness of."

"I have affirmations posted throughout the house that say, I CHOOSE LIFE," I say meaningfully.

"You are choosing life." Chetana nods her head in agreement. "Just because you want it. Spirit says, My Child of Light, you are blessed and will be healed. You will live a long and healthy life."

"That's both wonderful and comforting to hear," I say moved to tears. "And this information from Spirit makes sense to me. Even my birth was questionable, and when I was born

A YEAR OF MIRACLES

I almost died. As an infant and young child, I almost died a number of times. And as an adult I had two close calls with death. In my near death experience at thirty five, I came back for my children. But this time it's for me, because I Choose Life. I choose to live a long, healthy, happy, productive life, experiencing the love and joy in my relationship with Stan, my children, my family and friends. And of course God," I add reverently.

"You have been healing from infancy on," Chetana says lovingly. "The major focus of this lifetime is on healing, and helping others heal. At some point, you will share this healing journey of yours. You will become a beacon of Light for many. You will shine, and attract attention. Those who need your Light will find you, and you will help them heal."

"I believe that," I reply, feeling humble and awed. "I believe that with all my heart."

"Spirit has another message for you," Chetana adds. "Spirit says treat your body kindly. Be a loving parent to it. Nurture it, as if it is your beloved child. Tell it often what a good job it is doing. Praise it and thank it for working so hard. When you love and appreciate your body, and let it know that you do, your body will respond to your praise."

"I am already doing that," I say. "I really believe my body is doing a very fine job. I'll make sure to continue to praise it frequently."

"Do you have any questions for Spirit?" Chetana asks.

"Just one. Stan and I will be married July 12th. We believe I will be healed by then. What does Spirit say?"

Chetana falls silent, listening intently.

I sit watching her, holding my breath.

"You will be completely healed by your wedding day," she replies. "I am surprised Spirit has given me such a direct answer to a specific date. That is highly unusual."

I take a deep breath, and begin to breathe again.

A smile spreads slowly across Chetana's face, as she turns towards me.

"Spirit has just informed me that the unequivocal 'Yes' is because you know there is work to do, and you will follow through and do it. Spirit says you will do what it takes to heal."

On January 15th, I am sitting with Dr. Chang and his assistant Bob in a conference room at the University of Michigan Medical Center. I am reading a four page, single spaced, informed consent form which I need to sign. Once I sign the consent form, the vaccination of my irradiated cancer cells and BCG into both my thighs can begin. I am familiar with the protocol and possible side effects from my work with James, and reading about them does not provoke undue anxiety. Not until I come to the part that stops me dead in my tracks, and brings on the fear.

> "Your tumor has spread to the point where such usual cancer treatments as surgery, radiation therapy, hormonal therapy, and chemotherapy will not cure your disease. These forms of treatment have limited effectiveness in selected cases of advanced cancer. You are being offered participation in a study to test a new treatment involving the use of your lymphocytes, also called white blood cells, which are 'sensitized' to react to, and hopefully kill, your tumor. It is not possible to say whether or not you will benefit from the use of this therapy, but knowledge may be gained that will benefit others. If your disease becomes worse during the treatment program, you will be informed. The purpose of the treatment is to:
>
> 1) determine the side effects of the treatment, and to
> 2) determine how beneficial the treatment is in your situation. As this is a new therapy, side effects which may cause your condition to deteriorate, may be encountered. You will be watched closely for any side effects."

Icy spasms of fear, race up and down my spine, as the dumb, deformed giant shuffles into the room, and heads straight for the empty chair next to me.

"I'm back," he says grinning, his sour breath hot on my face. "I gotchya now."

"No," I say. "Go away. It was only a momentary lapse."

The giant looks confused. "Huh?" he says, scratching his head.

"I'm not afraid of you. Get lost."

"Boo," he shouts, lunging at me.

"OUT," I yell, in my most authoritative voice. "GET OUT OF HERE THIS MINUTE."

The giant sizes me up, realizes he can't frighten me, and shuffles slowly out the door.

I breathe a sigh of relief.

"Where do I sign?" I ask Dr. Chang. "Let the healing begin."

As the vaccination is readied, I visualize floating in my, by now, familiar pond. I lie there peacefully, completely surrounded by tall cedar trees. A cone of sunlight filters through the small opening in the circle of trees, and focuses on my thighs. I lie in the cool water, the scent of cedar permeating the air, mindful of my breathing and the rise and fall of my abdomen.

As Dr. Chang injects the vaccination into my thighs, I feel the energy of the sun enter my body, and say silently to myself, "Enter and Heal." I see my immune system located in my groin area being stimulated, and I see killer cells and T cells being born in large quantities, to specifically fight and destroy the cancer cells. I lie there for the next ten minutes, intensely visualizing this sequence.

I will continue to do this visualization many times a day over the next ten days, until my lymph glands are removed from my groin, stimulated with the antibody OKT3 and IL2 in the test tube, and allowed to multiply for the next two to three weeks. Dr. Chang's research indicates that this potent combination may be able to train my lymphocytes to recognize and attack the cancer cells in my body. I am counting on it, for I have added an especially unique ingredient to the potent mixture. It is a conditioned response that grows stronger each day, through my regular use of the immunotherapy tape.

As the days progress, so does my certainty that immunotherapy coupled with all I am doing, will be completely effective in ridding my body of cancer. The tumor is so small, my faith has grown so strong, and the treatment is so powerful, how could it be otherwise? I find myself knowing on a deep soul level that my life will never be as it was prior to the occurrence of cancer, and for this I am thankful. Although I would have preferred a different, easier, less life threatening way to fully and consciously choose life, that was not to be my path. The gifts I am receiving walking this path as a physical and spiritual being are treasures beyond any I can imagine.

I love who I am. All of me. My strengths and frailties. My light side, and my dark side. My very essence. I am learning much about love, forgiveness, and compassion. Towards myself. Towards others. I am developing a genuine acceptance of the authentic being that I am. I understand, regardless of how I would have preferred to learn, that choice in a very real sense was not mine to make. Divine Order decreed the form of the lesson. But the choice that remains mine, and determines my soul's growth, is how I respond, and what I learn from this teaching. I am pleased with who I am finding out I am.

I notice myself singing the Navakar Mantra frequently throughout the day. It has such a steadying influence on my life, this calling upon the Enlightened Beings who have overcome their inner enemies to help me overcome my inner enemies as well. In the evening Sharon stops by, and we walk into Brent's room to feed his hamsters Sue and Norm. Brent swears they are named after the cashier and manager at the movie theater where he works summers, but I don't believe him.

"Why would I name them after you and dad?" Brent innocently asks, a devilish grin spreading slowly across his face. "You've been divorced for years."

I could give him many reasons, but I keep quiet.

A YEAR OF MIRACLES

We find Sue, who was healthy and playful earlier in the day, listless and ill. I am fearful she is close to death. Norm runs around the cage frantically, clearly upset by this turn of events. I place Sue in the palm of my hand, and Sharon and I take turns holding and stroking her. We offer Sue treats, which she refuses, and gently wash her eyes, which are oozing pus and tightly shut. During the two hours that we minister to Sue, I sing the Navakar Mantra over and over. At the end of the evening, Sue is somewhat better, and within two days is fully recovered. I can't help but interpret this as a powerful omen. Sue recovering from a close encounter with death. The message couldn't be any clearer.

On January 24, 1992 I am back as an outpatient at the University of Michigan Medical Center, where three of my lymph nodes are removed from my groin under local anesthetic. It is obvious that Dr. Chang is extremely pleased upon removing them. He says the lymph nodes are fat and loaded with lymphoids. I think of them as sassy, and am convinced this is as a result of the imaging I have been faithfully doing.

Before I leave for home, my right arm is injected with irradiated cancer cells. This will help determine if my immune system is responding to, and attacking, cancer cells on its own. I am forewarned that there is not likely to be a reaction, but two days later the area is raised and red, showing my immune system is working to combat the cancer. In addition, the site of injection on both my thighs has become red, swollen, and ulcerated during these past ten days. As physically repugnant and painful as this area has become, it actually represents good news, because it indicates my immune system is strong and active. I am ecstatically happy, and thank and praise my immune system for the wonderful work it is doing. If I listen closely, I can hear my immune system responding to the praise by working even harder.

Immunotherapy is scheduled to begin February 6, 1992, and I sit at the computer writing the letter I will send to well over one hundred people, asking them to be part of my healing circle. Words come to mind effortlessly, and the letter almost writes itself. When I am finished, I read it over, pleased with what I have written.

Dear... ,

I am writing to ask you to take part in a healing circle of family and friends, who will be sending specific healing energies my way from February 6th through February 13th. At that time I will be at the University of Michigan Medical Center, receiving a new and very promising cancer treatment called immunotherapy. Immunotherapy involves the use of my own white blood cells, which are sensitized to react to and kill only my cancer cells, leaving my immune system intact. This is a very holistic approach, and one I feel quite comfortable with. During my stay in the hospital, I will receive sixteen thirty minute infusions intravenously, spaced eight hours apart, and here is where I would like your help.

I would like you to visualize these special cancer fighting cells doing three specific things.

1- See the cancer fighting cells surrounding the cancer cells and shooting special bullets into them, and the cancer cells leaking and exploding. I use the image of butterflies shooting bullets out of their antennae, but you can use any image that works for you.

2- See the cancer fighting cells dropping a substance on the cancer cells that causes them to dissolve. I see large rain clouds above the cancer cells opening and pouring rain on them, but again any image is fine.

3- See special scavenger cells come into the area and clean up the debris. My image is of elephants sucking the dead cells up with their trunks and carrying them away.

The tumor is very small, and is on my seventh left rib, fairly close to my spine. I find it helpful to focus my energies on that area when doing the imagery. I am in good spirits, and am feeling prepared, enthusiastic, and healthy. Recent tests show that my immune system is strong, and is already fighting the cancer. I expect this treatment, coupled with all I have been doing, to be completely effective. I believe that positive energy creates positive results, and that more is better than less. Therefore, the more people who join in, the stronger the energy field.

I want to thank you for your help, your love, your caring, and your prayers. I will be in touch with each and every one of you, to share the results of this group healing. I expect to let you know that I am free of cancer.

IN LOVE AND LIGHT,
Susan

I take the letter to Kinko's, where I have copies printed in lavenders, violets, and pinks, all colors I think of as warm, spiritual, and healing. Back home, I write the name of each recipient on each letter, and sign it. I address over one hundred envelopes, stuff the letters inside, and seal them. Licking more than one hundred love stamps, I paste them on the envelopes. On January 28, 1992, the day of my son Brent's twenty first birthday, I bless the letters, drive to the post office, and with an uplifted and expectant heart, send them on their way.

The phone awakens me from a sound sleep the morning before I am to enter the hospital. I grab for it, not wanting to awaken Stan. We have talked late into the night, and I am groggy from too little sleep, and too many words. The call is from Dr. Chang, and I am instantly alert. I glance at Stan, and notice he is listening intently to the conversation, an inquisitive look on his face.

"Good morning Susan," Dr. Chang begins.

"A good morning to you too," I reply, wondering why the call.

"I'm calling to postpone immunotherapy another week," Dr. Chang says, answering my unspoken question.

"Why?" I ask surprised.

"To grow more cancer fighting cells," Dr. Chang replies. "There is no accurate way to predict just how fast the cells will grow in the laboratory, and we need to grow a certain amount in order to make the vaccine. Delays occur frequently, and that is nothing to be concerned about."

"So you need additional cells to make the vaccine, and more time to grow them."

"That is correct," Dr. Chang replies.

I have become familiar with the nuances in Dr. Chang's voice, and I hear the excitement in his.

"The cancer fighting cells we have grown are extremely potent and toxic to the tumor," he continues. "They recognize the tumor, attach to it, and shoot their perforin bullets into it, killing the cancer."

"I never thought I'd be delighted to have a toxic part of me," I say, "but I am now."

Dr. Chang laughs. "I want to postpone immunotherapy until February 14th," he continues.

"Dr. Chang, that's Valentines Day. I'm an incurable romantic, and want to spend it with Stan. Could we schedule it for the following day?" I ask.

Dr. Chang laughs again. "All right," he agrees. "We'll schedule admission for the afternoon of the 15th, but it might be a day or two later."

"Agreed," I say. "That way I could attend the wedding of my friends Ron and Joan's daughter Laurie, whom I have known since she was a toddler."

"I have additional good news for you," Dr. Chang says sounding pleased.

"What's that?" I ask eagerly.

A YEAR OF MIRACLES

"I've just finished reviewing your most recent CAT scan, and it is unchanged from last month. There has been no new tumor growth."

"Thank God," I murmur, convinced the visualization I am doing is responsible for this state of affairs. I thank Dr. Chang, and hang up the phone.

Stan looks at me questioningly. "What?" he asks.

I promptly burst into tears.

"It's the best news ever." I am sobbing as I tell him.

Stan's face is a maze of emotions as he listens to me. Tears slide down his cheeks. As I finish speaking, we reach out and embrace. Holding one another, our mutual tears of joy intermingle. Clearly a bright future awaits us, for we have been truly blessed by a loving, compassionate God.

"I will need to make many calls, and send new letters out, with the changed treatment dates," I say, regaining a semblance of composure, "but it will be a true pleasure. In fact, it will be nothing less than a labor of love."

After talking on the telephone nonstop the past two hours, my voice sounds scratchy and hoarse. Moving to the computer, I begin writing the new letter that will be sent out with the last mail pickup of the day.

> Dear... ,
> I am writing to let you know of a change in dates of admission to the University of Michigan Medical Center. The rescheduled dates are February 15th through February 22nd, but this could possibly be delayed a few additional days. My doctor, has informed me delays of a week or two occur with amazing regularity. This is because there is no way to accurately predict how quickly the cancer fighting cells will grow in the laboratory, and a specific amount are required to make the vaccine that will be used in my treatment.
>
> The very exciting news I have to share is that the cancer fighting cells which were taken

from my body in January, are proving to be potent and extremely toxic against the cancer cells. They are doing what the butterflies do in my imagery... shooting bullets into the cancer cells and causing them to leak and explode. I personally believe this is due in part to the healing energies you have been sending my way. I am delighted to be entering treatment with a concrete affirmation that this vaccine is working against my cancer. I imagine the vaccine will be even more potent and toxic against the cancer once it is injected into my body. I have felt like an athlete in training for the Olympics these past few months. Now I am ready to win the Gold Medal.

Thank you for the imagery you have been doing. I am asking that you extend it through the end of February, so that a loving, healing circle of energy will be focused on me, before, during, and after treatment. The reason I have requested you work with three specific images is because they represent processes that actually take place during immunotherapy. However, any kind of healing energies you wish to send will be helpful and gratefully received.

Once again, thank you for your help, your love, your caring, and your prayers. I have both trust and faith that you will be hearing from me with the joyous news, that I am cancer free.

IN LOVE AND LIGHT,
Susan

What I have not given much thought to, is just how much it means to those in my healing circle to have an opportunity to actively participate in my healing. The letters that arrive daily tell a story I will always remember. They serve as a reminder of the importance of reaching out to others.

A YEAR OF MIRACLES

From Michael and Debbie:

You can count on us to be a committed link in your circle of healing. For our part we will be visualizing

1- black cancer cells shriveling up (like plants deprived of water) and withering away, like the passing of a season;

2- the Spirits of the Four Directions, especially the four white horses from the North, coming to turn the circle so that cancer cells are destroyed by the purifying power of the Native American's Spirits, and

3- the power of Nature restoring its environment, like in a lake, where poisons of the land are diluted and flushed away to the darkest regions of the deepest oceans.

Our prayers and thoughts are with you.

From Keriann:

Thank you for your letters, your visualizations, and above all, for reaching out to me and others. I hold you gently in my heart, and send loving, warm prayers.

From Barbara:

I received your letter about your upcoming immunotherapy, and it not only is a holistic approach, it is also a respectful way to work with the cancer cells. You can count on me, my prayers, and my visualization in accordance with the images you use. We will see one another in March in San Diego, and it will be an honor for me to meet your sweetheart.

From Dee Dee:

I want to let you know I'll be happy to do the visualizations. My normal meditation time is 6:00 a.m. on weekdays and a little later on weekends. Currently, I send Divine Light and Love enfolding you. For the time period you requested, I will do the visualizations, and thereafter will return to the Light and Love.

From Rose:

Like the Gray Wolf bonding to the family, you have bonded to life. My heart is open to send you energy during your treatments. I think of you often each day. May you dwell in the Light.

From Carolyn:

I have held a bird in my hand for a moment, a rainbow in my eyes for awhile, and you I'll hold in my heart forever. I have been imaging like crazy. The elephants are flying, and the butterflies have trunks!!!

From Kate:

Thank you for the opportunity to participate in your healing. It is an honor to be part of a powerful group of your friends, as we meditate upon your healing process. My love and positive energy are with you.

From Barbara and Bernie:

We are with you in your time of need. I am imaging you in a rose-gold glow. This week I will be in a seminar called, "Seeking the Feminine Divine," where we will be in frequent meditation. During those times, I will imagine a blue-violet aura going from my body into yours, with each breath I take.

From Elaine:

Thank you for allowing me to be part of your Healing Circle. I find it to be very rewarding. I really respect and admire the way you took responsibility for your own process, and then put people in place in a very strategic manner. Your faith in God, Susan, is a true inspiration for all. So many people wait for the law of the Doctor, instead of taking charge themselves. Good job my friend. Shalom.

From Melanie:

> Just wanted to let you know I've been visualizing for you. I believe you will be free of cancer. I think it is wonderful you are taking care of yourself, and healing in such an active way. It takes courage and strength. I also appreciate that you are able to ask for help.

It is letters like these that let me clearly see I am giving energy as well as receiving energy from those individuals who make up my Healing Circle. And in recognizing this Truth, I experience a profound connection with All That Is.

The week before immunotherapy speeds by. Marilyn, having made plane reservations based on my original treatment dates, arrives for a ten day stay February 8th. Stan and I pick her up at the airport, go out for dinner, and then return home. It is fitting to have Marilyn with me during these final days, as I prepare for immunotherapy. As always, she is upbeat and positive. We watch funny videos, laugh frequently, go clothes shopping for my upcoming March trip to San Diego, and just enjoy hanging out together. Stan and Marilyn have developed a special friendship of their own, and it is easy for the three of us to spend many happy hours together.

All my children tend to stop by often, but this week their comings and goings are noticeably accelerated. It seems every time I turn around, at least one of them is by my side.

"You're spoiling me," I say to Elyssa, as she hands me yet another sandwich from Zingerman's.

"Eat," my daughter insists, sounding like her mother. "You need to keep up your strength."

Obediently, I bite into the sandwich.

"Don't you have to study for midterms?" I ask Brent.

"Yeah," he grins wickedly, "but I'd rather visit with Sue and Norm."

"Good idea," I agree, laughing heartily.

"Josh and I dropped by just to sing for you," Tracy explains, and for the next half hour I am treated to a variety of show tunes.

"I'm here just because I want to be with you," Sharon says, direct and to the point.

"That's a good enough reason for me," I answer, happy for her company.

"I was just in the neighborhood, showing a house to a prospective buyer," Jennifer says in an offhand manner.

"Every day this week?" I innocently ask.

"She's a serious buyer," Jennifer replies with a straight face.

The phone, which is seldom silent, rings more frequently, as friends and family call, and with loving words wish me a complete healing. I can actually touch the loving energies surrounding me. A living, breathing presence fills my body, and directs my life in the most tender of ways.

February 13th Dr. Chang calls with the news that my admission has been changed from the afternoon of the 15th to the afternoon of the 16th of February. This pleases me, because now I will be able to attend Laurie's wedding, and be part of her celebration. There is another celebration I would like to attend on the 16th, so taking a deep breath, and figuring I have nothing to lose by asking, I do just that.

"Dr. Chang. Is it possible for me to check into the hospital that evening rather than that afternoon?"

"Whatever for?" Dr. Chang asks, sounding surprised.

"There is a small birthday party for my friend Marilyn early that evening," I say. "She has flown in from California to be with me, and I would like to attend."

"You would need to be here by 8:30 p.m. I want you completely prepared for your first treatment, which is scheduled for early Monday morning."

"I can do that," I say. "Thank you Dr. Chang. It really means a lot to me."

"You're welcome Susan. I'll expect you Sunday evening," he answers, kindness coloring his words.

A YEAR OF MIRACLES

Valentines Day, is all I ever dreamed it could be. Romantic. Sensual. Passionate. Loving.

"The first of many," Stan promises.

I nod and kiss his lips in agreement.

Beside being beautiful, Laurie's wedding is also life affirming. So many people I love are celebrating with her. All of my children. Many of my friends. Loved ones come and go, stopping by my side, wishing me well. I feel supported, surrounded and nurtured by love.

Stan and I dance heart to heart.

"The next wedding is ours," he whispers in my ear.

"I can hardly wait," I reply, visions of our wedding day dancing in my head.

"Same here," he murmurs as we twirl around the dance floor.

Early the following afternoon, Stan and I bring everything I will need to my room in the Cancer Care Research Unit at the University of Michigan Medical Center.

An hour later, the antiseptic, impersonal room has been changed into one that is cheery, welcoming, and a reflection of me. My mood is relaxed and serene. Having done all I know to prepare myself, and trusting in the goodness of God, I am at peace. I look forward with great anticipation to immunotherapy. But, for now, there is a party to attend.

The birthday party for Marilyn, hosted by her brother Bob and his wife Lynn is small and intimate. Marilyn's mother, Evalyn, has flown in from Chicago for the occasion. Marilyn's young niece and nephew, a few close friends, and Stan and I are present. After a gourmet dinner and delicious birthday cake, I hand Marilyn her gift. She opens it, admires it, and hugs me tightly.

"I'll be thinking of you constantly during this next week," Marilyn says, tears filling her expressive blue eyes.

"I know you will," I say softly, "and I draw strength from that."

"You're going to do it, Sue. You are going to heal completely."

"I know," I agree, nodding my head. "I really know I am."

"I love you, my soul sister," she whispers.

"And I, you," I whisper in return.

We stand side by side, fingers entwined, until Stan walks over, gently takes my arm, and lovingly guides me out the door. The most profound adventure of my life is about to begin. Having completed three months of intensive training, at long last I am going for the Gold.

A YEAR OF MIRACLES

CHAPTER 19

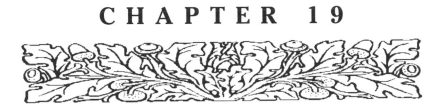

Going for the Gold

My hospital room is as welcoming as such a room can ever be. Filled with my most personal and beloved possessions, I experience my room as a calm oasis in a sea of anonymity and sterility. My butterfly quilt and sheets serve as a continual reminder of the healing butterflies of my imagery. My personal healing crystals lying on the bedside table radiate powerful energy throughout the room. Photographs of those I love line the window ledge, and my favorite pictures hang on the walls. The overall sensory feeling is one of empowerment, love, and hope. It is a fitting room for the manifestation of miracles.

I have barely settled into the room, when Elyssa and Jeff enter.

"Nothing from Zingerman's tonight. Just us," Elyssa smilingly says. "We were in the neighborhood."

"Right," I answer, delighted they stopped by.

The phone rings continuously for the next hour and a half.

"It's just like being at your house where the phone is never silent," Stan grumbles.

I laugh out loud.

"I feel so well loved," I respond happily. "Elyssa, Jeff, and you are here with me now. Sharon and Chuck, Pat, Marilyn, Brent, and Susan, all calling at the eleventh hour. It's such a wonderful gift of love to receive."

"It is," Stan agrees. "I'm just sounding grumpy because I'm feeling nervous. I don't want you to experience pain of any kind. Sometimes, it's hard to watch you go through difficult things, even though I know this treatment will work."

"It's hard on all of us," I reply. "On me, and on those who love me."

"But it's worth it," Jeff declares, "because of the end results."

Four heads nod in solemn agreement.

An hour later the door to my room opens, and a young resident holding a catheter enters.

"Hello," he says cheerfully. "I'm here to insert this catheter into your chest wall. That way, the infusions can drip directly into the catheter, and we can avoid continuously poking you."

"Will it hurt?" I ask, suddenly feeling nervous.

"Not much," he answers. "I will numb the area around your chest wall with a local anesthetic, so you won't feel the catheter as it enters. All you will feel is some pressure while I insert it, and some soreness for a few days afterwards."

"I can handle that," I say. "It sounds manageable."

"It ought to be," he agrees smiling at me. "Do you prefer the catheter on the right side or the left side?"

I answer without hesitation. "The tumor is on the left side, so insert the catheter on the left side. That way the infusions won't have as far to travel to reach the site of the tumor."

The procedure goes smoothly, and without incident. The catheter is inserted on the very first try, which, according to the resident, is highly unusual. Alone in my room I meditate, waiting for the night to pass and for my first treatment to begin.

In meditation I am talking to my tumor, something I have been doing these past few weeks.

"I know you are getting ready to leave," I affirm. "Perhaps you are even gone by now. I hope you are, for it would be easier on you to have transmuted. This treatment is very powerful and will destroy you."

I listen for a response, but hear only silence.

"If you are still here," I continue, "I hold you in the Light, and ask that you be transformed into healthy cells. Or, if you prefer, may you dissolve into the Light and move on in peace."

Still no answer.

"I bless you, and release you," I conclude. "And I thank you for the lessons you have taught me. I have learned them well, and they will remain a part of me for all the days of my life."

I do not know I am crying until I feel the tears as they slide down my cheeks.

"I'm doing it," I think. "It is happening right now. Tonight is the beginning of this phase of my treatment. Along with everything else I have been doing, this experimental immunotherapy protocol is what I am counting on to heal from cancer. No wonder I feel so emotional. So very much is riding on this."

I catch the tears on my tongue, and swallow them, enjoying their salty taste. Coming out of meditation, and feeling in harmony with All That Is, I swiftly fall into a dreamless sleep.

I have nothing but the highest of praise for the nursing staff that cares for me. They truly deserve the title "Angels of Mercy," for they are warm, caring, encouraging, compassionate, and inquisitive. Many of the nurses question me on the alternative methods I have been using, and see value in them. They are eager to help me implement my program in whatever way they can. When the nursing staff learns that I need an hour prior to the infusion, and half an hour during the infusion to meditate and visualize, it is duly noted on my chart. During the following week, day or night, a nurse enters my room an hour prior to my treatment, reminding me to begin my healing program. While I meditate and visualize, a sign is hung outside of my door. It reads, "Treatment In Progress. Keep Out." The entire nursing staff vigilantly takes steps to enforce this message. I soon discover that every nurse in the Cancer Care Research Unit is committed to being an ally in my healing. I will always be grateful for the support, encouragement, and loving care they lavish upon me during this most crucial period of time.

"What is that?" I ask Grace, pointing to the thick plastic bag filled with clear liquid she holds in her hand.

"Those are your LAK cells," Grace answers. "Are you ready to begin immunotherapy?"

"You bet I am. I'm ready to kick ass, and be done with this cancer once and for all."

Grace laughs out loud and continues talking.

"'I'm hanging the bag on the pole by the side of your bed, and hooking it to your IV. Then I will start the drip, and the LAK cells will enter your body. The complete infusion will take about thirty minutes, and no one will be allowed in your room during that time. But during the last five minutes I will come in to squeeze the bag and make sure all the LAK cells enter your body. I will try not to disturb you."

"Will you or another nurse come in five minutes before the end of every treatment?" I ask.

"Yes," Grace answers, "but as unobtrusively as possible. We all respect what you are doing."

"That won't be a problem," I respond. "As long as I know what to expect, I'll be able to incorporate it into my visualization."

I look closely at the bag. This nondescript liquid contains my altered white blood cells, which have been sensitized to react to and kill the cancer cells. Weeks of painstaking laboratory procedure reside within that bag, just as months of intensive imagery, hope, trust, faith and prayers reside within me. There is a ritual I need to do to mark this sacred moment. But lying in a hospital bed hooked up to an IV, a catheter inserted in my chest, my options appear limited.

"Grace, I want to hold the bag," I say.

Grace peers at me intently, and transfers the bag to my outstretched hands.

I close my eyes and say a silent prayer. "God, I trust in You as the source of all good. I am praying in faith, knowing You are blessing these LAK cells, and sending them on their journey to help heal me of cancer. Thank You for the good You are sending my way."

Opening my eyes, I hand the bag to Grace, watching as she swiftly hooks it onto the pole.

"I'm praying for your complete recovery," Grace says, as she begins the infusion, and quietly walks out of my room.

I push the play button on my tape recorder, and the familiar immunotherapy tape begins. Lying in the hospital bed, visualizing as I have done so many times before, I can actually feel the live LAK cells, envisioned as Divine White Light, entering the catheter, and coursing through me in search of cancer cells. It feels quite similar to the rehearsed imagery, yet as I tune in to my body, there is no way to mistake the subtle differences between the imagined and the real LAK cells. I hear the LAK cells buzzing with Divine Energy. Somewhat like a low, constant, soothing melodic hum. In my mind's eye, I see LAK cells converging at, surrounding, and covering the tumor, until all that is visible is a large circle comprised of Divine White Light. A smaller number of LAK cells are periodically sent out on patrol to search for stray cancer cells, but quickly return to rejoin the expanding Circle of Light. I perceive this as an affirmation that the cancer is located only on my seventh rib, and nowhere else.

I relax into the bliss of the Light as it travels through my body. I am completely embraced by the Light, both inwardly and outwardly. I know if I were to open my eyes, the whole room would be filled with Divine White Light, but I continue to keep them closed. I feel myself surrendering to the Light, as it flows through me, healing my body, my mind, and my soul.

I am finishing a late lunch when Dr. Chang walks into the room.

"How is it going, Susan?" he asks, checking the catheter.

"So far so good," I answer. "I had the LAK cell infusion early this morning, followed by the first Interleukin 2 treatment immediately afterwards. The only problem is that someone checks my vital signs every two hours. I'm going to end up sleep deprived."

Dr. Chang laughs and nods his head in agreement. "It certainly is disruptive, but this is a very potent treatment, and it is crucial to make sure you don't experience dangerous side effects," he explains. "That is why you are being monitored so frequently."

"I understand," I reply. "It will just take some getting used to. Perhaps I'll develop the knack of sleeping through it."

"If you continue tolerating the treatment, we will up your dosage to eighteen Interleukin 2 infusions from the fifteen originally planned," Dr. Chang says.

"When will we know?"

"Within the next day or two," Dr. Chang replies.

"I'll tolerate it," I say. "My body experiences this treatment as a healing one, and will welcome the Interleukin 2 infusions."

"I believe you could be right about that," Dr. Chang smilingly agrees. "It would not surprise me at all."

It is almost midnight. Having just finished my third Interleukin 2 treatment, I am listening to a Bob Dylan tape when Stan enters the room. He is carrying a large picture in his arms.

"I've worked on this all day," he says kissing me soundly, "and finally it's finished."

"What is it?" I ask curiously. "Don't keep me in suspense."

Stan turns the picture around. Inside the frame is a collage of photographs of large, strikingly beautiful, exotic butterflies.

"How absolutely perfect," I say, touched by the multitude of ways Stan has of demonstrating his love.

Stan grins. "I must have searched through at least fifty Michigan Natural History magazines, collecting the most beautiful butterflies to include in this collage."

"I can't think of a more loving and appropriate gift, Stan," I exclaim.

"I couldn't either," Stan agrees. "That's why I created it for you."

"Thank you," I say softly. "I am the luckiest woman alive."

Stan laughs. "I won't argue with that," he says, as we kiss again.

"You've had four treatments without side effects, and are tolerating the treatments well," Dr. Chang says smiling, and sounding pleased. "I'm optimistic that you will be able to complete eighteen treatments, instead of the original fifteen."

I smile back, happy that I am doing so well, and anticipate this good fortune continuing. The work James and I have done is paying off, and it appears the toxic side effects of Interleukin 2 will remain minimal.

"Thank you James," I silently intone. "Your assistance has been invaluable, and your name will be printed throughout the book I am committed to writing. I want more people to learn about the work you do, and see it as a valuable complementary treatment."

Coming out of my reverie, I turn to Dr. Chang, and ask him the question that has been continuously on my mind.

"How quickly will the tumor dissolve?" My voice is strong and confident.

"There will not be an instantaneous regression," Dr. Chang responds. "At the end of the month, there may be some shrinkage in the tumor, and at the end of two months, some additional changes may take place. If the tumor completely dissolves, it is likely to occur over an extended period of time."

Disappointment wraps itself around me, squeezing all the joy out of my body.

"Oh," I say in a flat dull voice, and fall silent.

After Dr. Chang leaves, I replay our conversation, think about it, and arrive at a decision. Despite Dr. Chang's expectations, I will hold to my own vision. I will continue visualizing the tumor dissolving. Completely gone from my body at the end of this treatment. In addition, I will envision the CAT scan that is scheduled a month from now showing no trace of cancer anywhere in my body. I realize my vision may not happen, but until shown otherwise, I will hold firmly to a complete and permanent healing.

My approach to healing is significantly different from the majority of cancer patients, given the alternative healing methods I freely make use of. And certainly it is to my advantage that the lesion is small and localized. Although I don't consider myself a gambler, I would wager that I will fully respond to this treatment, and that my uniqueness will play a large and significant part in my recovery. Fully embracing this decision with mind, body, and spirit, the heaviness of disappointment dissolves, as the lightness of joy reenters my body.

A YEAR OF MIRACLES

With each additional treatment the butterflies in my imagery multiply. As far as the eye can see, and beyond, they are everywhere. Large, colorful, powerful butterflies. Mostly monarchs, their bright orange bodies outlined in black, glistening in the Light. I am enraptured. Enchanted. Mesmerized by their beauty and grace. Treatment by treatment, they grow more beautiful, more powerful, more abundant.

After eight treatments I am restless and bored. There is some water retention and redness, but it is minimal. Both the doctors and nursing staff voice surprise and delight over how well I am tolerating the treatment. Physically, I feel much too healthy to be in the hospital, where there isn't enough to keep me occupied. Sleeping seems like a distant memory, with my vital signs being monitored every two hours, day and night. I exercise by walking up and down the corridors of the 7th floor, my IV pole trailing behind me, and I have become a familiar presence at the gift shop on the second floor. I read until my eyes grow bleary, and have even gotten desperate enough to watch some television. Mornings and evenings I meditate and sing malas. Throughout the day I wander around the room, looking at photographs, and inhaling the fragrance of flowers that transform my room into a floral delight. The red roses from Stan sit in a vase on the bedside table. I smell them often, and day dream about the man I love.

My mother had a saying I did not like, though I never told her so.
"All good things must come to an end," she would occasionally state.
It happens today late in the afternoon.

After my tenth treatment, my unblemished record of tolerating the Interleukin 2 without side effects ends abruptly. Within minutes after completing the treatment, I find myself chilled to the bone. I ring for additional blankets which I burrow under. They prove useless in keeping me warm. Feeling unabashedly miserable and running a fever, I shiver uncontrollably under the pile of blankets. Nausea forces me to a sitting position, and I violently heave breakfast and lunch into a waiting bedpan. For the rest of the day I remain in bed dozing intermittently, unaware of having my vital signs monitored.

Feeling better the following day, I become aware an old childhood tape has been triggered by my adverse reaction to the treatment.

"The reason you reacted badly is because you were talking to family and friends about how well you were doing," the childhood voice says accusingly.

"That's ridiculous," I adamantly reply.

"No, it's not," the voice insists. "Don't you remember? You should never give yourself a 'cunnuh hurra.'"

Now I remember the old Jewish superstition I was raised with. Don't ever acknowledge something good is happening to you. Because if you do, the evil eye, ear, nose, throat, or mouth, is going to see it, hear it, smell it, taste it, or speak it, and turn something good into something bad. This is expressed in Jewish shorthand as, "Don't give yourself a cunnuh hurra."

"It's only an old superstition," I say, "and besides, it's not true. The reason I had the reaction is because bodies respond this way to Interleukin 2. Most patients have this reaction during their second infusion, and for sometime after. Other patients can't complete a full course of treatment, because it is too hard on their systems. But this was my tenth, and since then I've had two more. I'm feeling good again. I'm two thirds of the way there, with only six more treatments to go, and I'm proud and excited."

"So just play it safe for now," the voice pleads. "Don't do anymore cunnuh hurras. Agreed?"

I laugh out loud, and answer. "No deal. If I give in to you on this, it won't stop there. I grew up with too many superstitions, and you always are there to remind me of them."

"I just want things to go well for you."

Listening closely, I hear the words of a frightened, superstitious, innocent, young girl.

"I know you do. We both agree on that," I say soothingly. "I also want things to go well. And they will. Just trust me on this one, and you'll see for yourself."

The voice falls silent, but it is not convinced.

After my fourteenth treatment, my body breaks out in a massive head to toe rash. I itch terribly, and tear fitfully at my skin. The medication I receive does little to relieve the itching, and I am reminded of the time I suffered through a bad case of poison ivy. The fact that I am bloated with 15 pounds of extra fluid does nothing to improve my humor. Nor does looking in the mirror, and seeing a face I barely recognize. I was forewarned my skin might become extremely dry and flaky, and it has. Especially under the eyes, where I have developed wrinkles and bags that make me look like I imagine my future self might some thirty years from now.

"I want to live to grow old," I whimper to Grace who has brought me a thick white salve to apply, "but I didn't bargain on it happening overnight."

"It's only temporary, but I understand your feelings," Grace replies empathetically, one woman to another.

"If this is only a temporary price for the kind of healing I anticipate, it is a very small price to pay, but I must be vainer than I thought, because I hate looking like this," I admit.

"Don't be too hard on yourself for feeling that way," Grace says, a smile on her lips. "I don't know of any woman who wouldn't be bothered by such a drastic change."

I smile back at her with dried, cracked lips, feeling understood and validated.

"I threw up my dinner," I tell Stan, amazed and grateful that he is not repulsed by my physical appearance. "But I think it may have been more from what I ate, than from the treatment."

"What did you have?" he asks curiously.

"It sounds like a terrible combination, but it tasted good at the time."

"Tell me," he coaxes.

"I had pineapple juice, cream of broccoli soup, and chocolate milk," I answer somewhat defensively.

"You're pulling my leg," Stan insists. "What did you really have?"

"I just told you," I reply, feeling miffed.

"No wonder you heaved it up. Your stomach was much too smart to keep it down," Stan says, bent over in laughter.

"What's so funny?" Brent asks, coming into the room, followed by Elyssa, Tracy, and Sharon.

"Your mothers dinner," Stan says.

"Why?" all four ask simultaneously.

"Oh no," I moan, pulling the covers over my head.

Sunday morning I have my last Interleukin 2 treatment. Number eighteen, which is a magical number that represents Life in Judaism. When it is finished, I enter into meditation, giving thanks for the completion of this phase of my healing. I am so excited to be leaving the hospital. To have the catheter removed from my chest. To be unhooked from all machines. To sleep through the night in my own bed, without having my vital signs monitored. To spend the night in Stan's arms again. I feel fortunate this treatment was available to me, but I am more than ready to resume life outside the Cancer Care Research Unit at the University of Michigan Medical Center.

It is amazing how much there is to bring home. With everything packed, it looks like we will need a moving truck in order to clear out of here. When the door opens I turn expecting to see Stan, but it is Dr. Chang and his assistant Bob who enter the room.

"I see you're leaving us," Dr. Chang says by way of greeting.

"Actually, I'm looking forward to it. Nothing personal," I respond.

"Your CAT scan is scheduled for March 26th at 8:00 a.m.," Dr. Chang says, "and I'll see you March 30th at 1:00 p.m. to discuss the results. I'm feeling positive about this treatment."

"I expect the cancer to be gone," I say matter-of-factly.

"I would like that," Dr. Chang replies. "But remember, that may not be the case."

A YEAR OF MIRACLES

"My reality is that the cancer is gone," I silently remind myself. "Unless shown otherwise, that is the only reality I will continue to perceive."

After Dr. Chang leaves, Bob remains to fill out the discharge papers.

"The first month usually doesn't show much, but you can be different if you want," Bob says, a wonderful smile warming his face.

"I definitely want to be different," I immediately reply. "I'm planning on it. This is a blessed time in my life, a time to remember with gratitude and thankfulness. I trust in God's love, Bob. I know I am healed."

Bob gives me a hug. "I will pray for you," he says softly. "I will pray for a complete healing."

The door opens and Stan walks in. "Ready to split this joint?" he asks, kissing me soundly.

"About as ready as I'll ever be," I reply, envisioning a beautiful future spreading out before us, filled with an abundance of health, happiness, and never ending love.

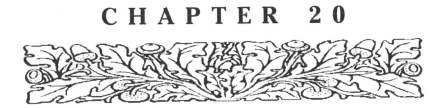

CHAPTER 20

And Now for the Good News

Only after I am home do I fully realize how much the treatment has taken out of me. I am physically exhausted, my energy level is depleted, and I spend the next week either sleeping, or sprawled on the couch resting. For the first time, I personally experience the meaning of the term "couch potato." In my naiveté, I have scheduled clients, but there is no way I can honor this schedule, for I need more time to build up my strength. The disability insurance policy I bought ten years ago proves a financial blessing, assuring a steady income when I am unable to work. Once again, I thank my insurance agent who had the persistence to convince me that a self employed single woman could not afford to be without this protection.

After two weeks, I feel more like myself, and shortly thereafter Stan and I leave for California to participate in Gwen's week long intensive healing workshop. The timing could not be more opportune, for my body delights in trading cold, snow, and sleet, for warmth, sunshine, and the Pacific Ocean. I notice an immediate difference in my energy level, and spend as much time as I can outdoors, remembering to honor my body by giving it the frequent periods of rest it still needs.

Being with Gwen is a gift I give myself gladly, for I grow, learn, and heal on an ever deepening level when in her presence.

A YEAR OF MIRACLES

"You are my miracle child," Gwen says, embracing me by way of greeting, and I know she speaks the truth.

To add to my delight, Stan can now get to experience the beauty of Gwen, and the magic she weaves. Two years earlier on another intensive with Gwen, I pledged in a sacred ceremony to study the element of Fire for three years, three months, three weeks, and three days. As part of the ceremony, I had decorated a prayer arrow with fabric, crystals, feathers, and shells. Imbuing it with my heartfelt wishes and desires, I planted it overlooking the ocean in a secluded grove at Torrey Pines State Park. Barely a year later, my initiation by fire began, consuming all that was extraneous, cleansing, restructuring, and transforming my very life. But like the mystical Phoenix that consumes itself in flame, I have risen from the ashes of what some call fate, and been reborn again. Reborn into wholeness. Reborn into whom I am meant to be.

Gwen has a favorite spot at Torrey Pines, and it is here we hold a memorial service for Eyvor, a member of the group who died from melanoma three months ago. It is a fitting and moving tribute to a friend who exhibited both courage and serenity throughout her long illness. I flash back to the final time I saw Eyvor, a month before her death. Mostly I remember her face, how radiant and serene it looked. Eyvor was waiting to be discharged from the hospital. From there she would travel to her daughter's home, where she planned to die in the presence of those she loved most. Her husband. Her children. Her grandchildren.

I had just come from the CAT scan that would show the recurrence of cancer, and I have brought Eyvor a rose quartz crystal energized by our group. Eyvor reaches for it eagerly, her eyes aglow.

"Thank everyone in the group and tell them how moved I am by their show of love."

Her voice is low, as she strokes the crystal, and I strain to hear her.

"We'll miss you Eyvor," I say, tears springing to my eyes. "I wish the experimental immunotherapy had worked for you."

Eyvor stretches out her fingers, and wipes the tears from my eyes. "I'm ready. It's my time and I know it. I am truly at peace." Eyvor stares at me intently, and I feel her eyes boring into my soul. "But it's not your time. Not for a long time. Promise me, you won't forget that." Her voice rings strong with conviction.

"I promise Eyvor," I say, unaware of how my life is about to change.

The singing of "Amazing Grace" envelops me, and I am swiftly returned to the present.

"Sometimes I forget Eyvor," I silently admit, "but then I hear your voice and I remember again."

As I join in the singing, a sudden gust of wind lifts the hair off my face. It lingers for a moment, before disappearing as suddenly as it arrived. I recognize that Eyvor's playful spirit has joined us as we say our good-byes.

This week, in a special ceremony, Stan pledges to study the element of Earth. His pledge is joyously witnessed by the entire group. We form a circle around Stan, and pledge to support and honor him in this undertaking. Afterwards, Stan and I walk to a high bluff in Torrey Pines overlooking the majestic Pacific Ocean. We select a secluded and sheltered spot, and Stan takes the exquisite prayer arrow he has decorated, and plants it firmly in the earth. I plant a prayer arrow symbolizing the renewal of my pledge to Fire alongside it. Joining hands we create our own ceremony. Taking turns, we ask that God bless us with an abundance of love, laughter, and longevity. We ask God to be ever-present in our lives. To show us the way. To be our guiding light. To help us grow in goodness. To watch over our children and loved ones. We repeatedly thank God for the miracles already present in our lives, and dedicate ourselves to living life fully, and honoring the miracles still to unfold.

A YEAR OF MIRACLES

Stan then recites the following two prayers:

> *Bless us, dark earth as we give back*
> *that which we have received*
> *as we make a forest of blessing a ridge of blessing*
> *for the future to grow upon.*

Chinook Psalter

> *Hail Mother, who art the earth,*
> *Hallowed be thy soil, rocks, and flora that nourish*
> *   and support all life.*
> *Blessed be thy wind that gives us breath and thy*
> *   waters that quench, bathe, and refresh all living*
> *   things.*
> *Holy Earth... as one... we praise your majesty,*
> *   grace and wonder.*

Bill Faherty

Connecting with the fire energy, I recite this Masai Prayer:

> *Thank you Father for your free gift of fire.*
> *Because it is through fire that you draw near to us*
> *   every day.*
> *It is with fire that you constantly bless us.*
> *Our Father, bless this fire today.*
> *With your power enter into it.*
> *Make this fire a worthy thing.*
> *A thing that carries your blessing.*
> *Let it become a reminder of your love.*
> *A reminder of life without end.*
> *Make the life of these people to be baptized like*
> *   this fire.*
> *A thing that shines for the sake of people.*
> *A thing that shines for your sake.*
> *Father, heed this sweet smelling smoke.*
> *Make their life also sweet smelling.*
> *A thing sweet smelling that rises to God.*
> *A holy thing.*
> *A thing fitting for you.*

AND NOW FOR THE GOOD NEWS

Fingers intertwined, we stand silently, feeling the awakened energies of this sacred space swirling about us. With a last, lingering, backward glance at the two prayer arrows gently swaying in the breeze, we slowly retrace our steps, and rejoin our group of friends.

The day of leave taking, we gather on the windswept beach for a closing ceremony. I look around the circle at old and new friends. Familiar faces look back at me. Gwen. Stan. June. Betty. Anne. Dee Dee. Elaine. Joan. Barbara. Theresa. Anna. Kate. Glenn. Bernie. Gordon. Joseph. James. Faces turn towards me filled with love. Faces filled with belief in my healing. Faces that say I am blessed. I blink my eyes, imagining them to be a camera lens, and the picture is stored in my memory bank, preserving this moment forever.

It is never easy taking leave of people I love, and this time is no exception. Saying goodbye to June is by far the most difficult. No matter how long between visits, the easy camaraderie, the deep abiding love, and the zany, irreverent humor we share, keeps us connected. Only physical distance separates us. The mental, the emotional, the spiritual connection, is as close as it ever was. Knowing that June and her husband Jerry will be at our wedding in July helps ease our good-byes, as does looking forward to spending the next few days with Marilyn.

"There's the neatest shop in Santa Monica," Marilyn says, excitement coloring her voice," and I have a gut feeling your wedding dress is there."
"Your gut feelings are amazingly accurate. What are we waiting for?" I ask, my excitement matching hers.
Stan in tow, we set out for the mall.

"Wander about for awhile, and don't set foot in here," I say emphatically, pointing toward the store where Marilyn believes I will find my wedding dress.
Stan nods in compliance, and wanders off.
Marilyn and I eagerly enter the store, and systematically work our way through it. There are many beautiful dresses,

but none that call my name. Not until I round a corner, and come to a sudden halt. Spotlighted on a rack is a romantic, feminine, spun concoction of fine creamy gauze, exquisite lace, satin ribbons, and tiny, pale pink satin flowers, that are artfully applied to the dress. The neckline is rounded, and elasticized, and can be worn either on or off the shoulders. The dress is fitted at the waist and encircled by a matching wide lace sash that emphasizes the tiered full skirt, which is trimmed with a whisper of delicate lace and satin ribbons. I stand there spellbound.

"I've found my wedding dress," I manage to call out, and Marilyn instantly appears at my side.

"It's gorgeous. Try it on," she insists.

I don't need additional urging, and soon find myself looking in a three way mirror, delighted with my reflection.

"Oh Sue," Marilyn says in a rush of emotion. "You look so beautiful. You'll take Stan's breath away."

As if on cue, we hear Stan's voice in the doorway of the shop.

"Stay out," Marilyn yells. "Your bride to be is trying on her wedding dress. Come back in an hour."

"He's gone," the saleswoman announces, as we let out a collective sigh of relief.

"Not only did we find my wedding dress," I jubilantly say to Stan, "but we also found Marilyn's maid of honor dress."

"So you have to pay attention to my gut feelings," Marilyn adds laughingly, "and I'm having one right now."

"What is it?" Stan asks, joining in the fun.

"My gut feeling says that you are going to take us out to dinner at my favorite Chinese restaurant."

"I wouldn't dare do otherwise," Stan says grinning, arms around us both. "Just lead the way."

Our plane touches down at Detroit Metro Airport the evening of March 24th, just thirty six hours prior to my CAT scan.

"You know," I say to Stan on the ride home, "I expect the scan will show I am completely healed from cancer."

"That's what I'm counting on as well."

"But there is the possibility that despite everything, it might not work out that way."

"I know that," Stan answers in a subdued tone.

"Then what about our plans, our hopes and all our dreams for the future?"

"We'll go forward with them. No matter what, I'm committed to you. You can count on me."

I reach out in the dark, and squeeze Stan's fingers, a lump forming in my throat.

"It's not like I expect bad news. I just needed to discuss it with you. If the unexpected happens, we'll handle it together."

"Always together," Stan promises. "That's what commitment means."

"Thank you God," I say for the thousandth time. "Thank you for sending me Stan, who teaches through being who he is, what unconditional love is about."

Lighting the 28 candles on Sharon's birthday cake, the evening of March 25th, I reflect upon the changes since her previous birthday. I vividly recall the paralyzing fear I felt a year ago, during that first CAT scan to determine the type of cancer I had, and how advanced it was. Now one year later, calm, trusting, and at peace, I await the CAT scan which I anticipate will show all traces of cancer to be gone.

"One year," I think. "A full cycle of time from start to finish. Now the season to harvest has finally arrived, and I am as ready as I will ever be."

Carrying in the cake, I glance at the circle of smiling faces congregated around the table.

"Blow out your candles, and make a wish Sharon," I urge.

Sharon laughs softly. "You know what my wish is Mom."

"It hasn't changed all year," Chuck adds, his arm encircling Sharon lovingly

"It's the same wish we all have," Tracy says.

Heads nod in agreement.

"It's a wish that will be coming true very soon," I promise, my voice tinged with emotion. "And the love and support I feel from you all, is a big part of the reason it will."

A YEAR OF MIRACLES

Thursday morning I awaken while it is still dark, for an hour of prayer and meditation prior to leaving for the hospital. "God," I pray, "I trust Your Goodness, Your Love, and Your Caring. I am free from worry and fear, knowing Your loving presence goes with me. Thank You for teaching me patience, for guiding me, supporting me, and loving me. I feel safe and secure in Your presence, as I prepare for this scan. Praying to You in faith, I know You are blessing me now."

During meditation, the words "prepare for opportunity disguised as loss," flash through my mind a number of times, followed by an image from the book, "I Choose Life." In this image the parents of Garrett Porter, a young boy with a malignant brain tumor, are being told the tumor has dissolved, and all that remains is a bit of calcification to mark where it had been. I am convinced the words and image have appeared as a sign that the "loss" refers to the loss of my tumor, and I will be pronounced cancer free.

I leave for the scan feeling a trust and faith stronger and more powerful than ever before. It remains with me throughout the scan, and while the radiologist checks the films. I never once look up from the table I am lying on. Eyes closed, I sing malas, my special healing crystal in my hand, until I am told I can leave. As I go about my day, the feelings grow in intensity, until my body pulsates rhythmically, one living, breathing vibration of faith and trust.

I dream I am pregnant and in labor, about to give birth to new life. Some dreams need interpretation, for their meaning is elusive, but this dream does not. Its meaning is exceedingly clear, and I am euphoric throughout the weekend.

Sunday night, I have another dream relating to my healing. I don't wish to offend gentle sensibilities, but there is no other way I can say it. I am outdoors, carrying a dark bag filled with shit over my left shoulder, and looking for a place to dispose of it. After a very long walk, up hills and down, I see two outdoor toilets, and people waiting in line. The toilet on the right has many people waiting, whereas the toilet on the left, has only three. I stand in the shorter line waiting my turn. When it comes, I dump the bag and its contents into the toilet, flush it down into the bowels of the earth and leave. Noticing another bag lying under an oak tree, and knowing it is meant for me, I sit with my back against the tree, and open the brightly colored bag. It is filled with a variety of gold and silver coins. There are predominantly American coins, but some Canadian coins are intermingled with them. I am particularly attracted to one large gold coin, with a picture of Queen Elizabeth celebrating her 25th anniversary. I hold the coin, and cry tears of joy, for I know I have been given the most precious of all gifts, that of a long and rich life.

Monday, I arrive an hour before my appointment with Dr. Chang. Making my way down the corridor to the hospital chapel, I open the stained glass doors and enter in silence. Seated in the front pew, I bow my head in prayer. A kaleidoscope of emotions erupt and are swiftly discharged, while my tears flow freely. After regaining a semblance of composure, I walk across the room and face the large Jewish Star of David that shares wall space with an equally large cross. Reverently placing my fingertips on the points of the star, I remain standing lost in contemplation.

Reading through the oversized book that patients, family members, and friends have written poignant, eloquent, heartfelt prayers into, I add mine.

"God," I write, "I commend myself to Thy tender mercies. Thy Will be done."

I sign my name, date it March 30th, and with one last backward glance, open the chapel door and retrace my steps down the corridor, to the moment I have been waiting for.

I am in the examination room with Dr. Chang's assistant Bob, who is drawing my blood, for additional tests.

"Where is Dr. Chang, Bob? I thought I was going to see him today."

"Dr. Chang is in surgery, and it's taking longer than anticipated," Bob says soothingly. "He hasn't forgotten about you, Susan. He'll be here as soon as he can."

"Have you seen the scan or the report?" I ask.

"I haven't," Bob admits, "but another doctor looked at it earlier today, and he thought it was about the same."

"That's not possible. I know the tumor is gone." I am completely factual.

"Four weeks is too soon for any significant change to occur." Bob is as factual as I am.

"Remember, at the hospital you told me I could be different if I wanted to?"

Bob nods in agreement.

"I told you I wanted to, and I am. I don't care what the other doctor thought. I know I am healed."

A young intern enters the room. He listens quietly, and as I finish he begins to speak. "I took a quick look at the scan, and I didn't notice any change in your rib either."

"Did you see any of the earlier scans?" I ask pointedly.

"No," he admits. "I haven't."

"Then you really don't have anything to compare this scan to, and you aren't in a position to judge it, are you?" I ask, feeling my irritation rising.

"I guess not," he mumbles, and bolts from the room.

"Nor are you Bob," I continue. "It's all hearsay."

I am in awe of how unshakable my faith and trust in a complete healing remains.

"Let's wait until we hear from Dr. Chang," I say, my irritation abated.

"Agreed." Bob holds out his hand. I take it, and shake it warmly.

"What if Dr. Chang says the tumor hasn't changed?" a small inner voice asks, as I wait for him.

"He won't say that."

"But what if he does?" The voice is persistent.

"I would be surprised and terribly disappointed," I admit. "Heartbroken really, but still grateful that the tumor hasn't grown."

"And then what?"

"And then I'll put together an even more rigorous program, and the next time the tumor will be gone."

The voice falls silent, as if it wants to believe me.

"But that scenario is not going to happen," I say in a strong, clear voice, "because the tumor is no longer there."

The door opens, and Dr. Chang, wearing surgical scrubs, his face fatigued, enters the room.

I grip my healing crystal tightly, as I turn quizzically towards him.

"I still haven't had a chance to study the scan Susan, but I've just finished reading the report."

"What does it say?" I ask, heart suddenly in my throat, as I wait for the words he speaks to ring sweet in my ears.

"The report says the rib is more sclerotic, which means there is some new bone growth, and less tumor mass," he replies sounding gratified.

"Then the tumor is gone." It is a statement.

"No, the report doesn't say that. It says there is more bone, and less tumor. That is in keeping with a partial shrinkage of the tumor. And that is very good news. I will study the scan tomorrow, then call to let you know what I find."

Dr. Chang smiles at me looking very pleased, and within that smile I can sense how dedicated a doctor he is, and how deeply he cares.

"And if you agree with the report?" I ask.

"Then we would wait four weeks, do another CAT scan, and admit you into the hospital for another week of treatment with Interleukin 2. Only this time we will double the dosage."

"I don't believe that will be necessary, Dr. Chang."

"Why not?" he asks, looking puzzled.

"Because tomorrow when you view the scan, the tumor will be completely gone."

Back in the Chapel, I turn my thoughts once again to God.

"I know this is a test of my faith and nothing more," I say, "for in my deepest of hearts, I know I am healed. Soon others will also know and rejoice with me."

Exuding an air of peace, I leave the Chapel, my faith firmly anchored in my partnership with God.

A YEAR OF MIRACLES

March 31st is a balmy day with a healthy hint of spring in the air. Both Mocha and I are eager to be outdoors before the weather changes, as Michigan weather is apt to do this time of year. At Saginaw Forest I unleash Mocha, and together we wander the sometimes gentle, sometimes steep rolling path. Mocha bounds ahead, sniffing secret dog smells, tail wagging ferociously, intoxicated with her new found freedom. An hour later our steps grow slower, our breathing more labored, and in mutual agreement we turn and head for home.

While filling Mocha's bowl with cold water, I see the light on the answering machine blinking. Pressing the play button I hear Dr. Chang's voice on the tape. Gripping the counter, I listen to his message.

"Susan, this is Dr. Chang. I just finished reviewing your CAT scan and it is very good news. It looks like the rib tumor has responded very nicely, and new bone formation is present. I reviewed the results with my assistant Bob, and if I don't speak with you today, he'll talk with you about them tomorrow. Take care."

Not speak with me today? Unthinkable. But I am puzzled by the message. I tap the play button, and listen to the message again. And again. And again.

"Dr. Chang, what are you telling me?" I ask out loud. "Yesterday you told me there was new bone formation, so that's old news today. Is the cancer gone? That's what I want to hear. And if it is, wouldn't you have said so on the message? Especially since you know that I believe I am healed."

I pace back and forth, my mind weighing and dissecting the message.

"Dr. Chang sounds pleased, and he said the tumor responded very nicely, so the tumor must be gone," I think happily.

"Then wouldn't he have said that?" the small inner voice asks.

"Not necessarily. He probably wants me to hear the news from him."

"But he said if he didn't speak with you today, Bob would talk to you tomorrow."

"He knows I'll call as soon as I pick up the message."

"You haven't called though. You've been too busy debating the meaning of his message these past few minutes."

"You're absolutely right, and the only way I'll know if Dr. Chang means what I think he means, is by talking with him directly."

I look at the clock. It is 3:33 p.m.. Dr. Chang must still be in his office. I walk into my bedroom, pick up my healing crystal, grip it tightly in my hand, and dial his office. His secretary Debbie puts me through immediately.

"Dr. Chang, this is Susan. I'm returning your call." My voice sounds breathless.

Dr. Chang, wastes no time in getting directly to the heart of the matter.

"Susan, it's the very best news. The tumor is not visible."

"It's gone!" I shout, my voice rising.

"It's gone," Dr. Chang replies, excitement coloring his voice.

"Thank You God," I say gratefully, my voice ringing loud and clear. "Thank You for this miracle. Thank You for my life."

And I promptly burst into tears.

"Dr. Chang, I love you." I am laughing and crying simultaneously.

"I am so happy for you," Dr. Chang responds jubilantly.

"It's gone. It's gone. It's gone." I chant gleefully. "The tumor is gone."

Dr. Chang laughs a low laugh. "It's gone," he agrees. "The written report grossly underestimated what has occurred. There is no visible sign of tumor. And new bone is forming on your rib, where the cancer had eaten it away."

"So where do we go from here?" I ask happily. "Now that the cancer is gone."

"I want you to repeat immunotherapy in early May. This time we will double the dosage of the Interleukin 2," Dr. Chang gently replies.

"Why?" I ask, both surprised and puzzled. "I thought when the tumor was gone, the treatment would be completed."

"For two important reasons," Dr. Chang states thoughtfully. "If there are any stray cancer cells in your body, the Interleukin 2 will destroy them."

"Sort of like an insurance policy," I say speculatively.

"Exactly," Dr. Chang concurs.

"And the other reason?"

"The Interleukin 2 will help train your immune system to grow stronger through increased production of the specific cancer fighting cells."

"A double insurance policy," I think, and then speak out loud.

"I trust you Dr. Chang, and I'll do as you ask. But I don't want to dwell on that right now. I need to share this wonderful news with Stan, my children, my family and friends. I want to celebrate being cancer free."

"Enjoy your celebration. You certainly have earned it," Dr. Chang says warmly, and we say our good-byes.

"Please be home," I pray dialing Stan's number, and as God would have it, he is.

"You have to come over Stan. Right now. I have news."

I suspect that I sound bossy, but I am not overly concerned. I just want to be with Stan. To look into his expressive brown eyes when he hears the miraculous news, and to rejoice together.

"I'm on my way," Stan answers, hearing the urgency and excitement in my voice, and within minutes he races into the house.

I don't remember the exact words I use, nor does Stan. Nevertheless, I will remember forever the exquisite look of joy on Stan's face, as my fingertips trace the tears flowing freely down his cheeks. As we embrace, two hearts beating as one, our life together stretching before us, the road ahead long and wondrous, the gift of time to live out our dreams a reality, I feel a quickening in my body, and know at last, I am healed and whole.

EPILOGUE

Living the Miracle

Glancing out the window of my study, preparing to write the final pages of this book, the lush green beauty, new growth, and profusion of life in our yard profoundly affects me. A carpet of tightly clustered violets forms a ground cover in which squirrels romp, while a family of brightly colored purple finches sings melodiously as they fly from nest to tree, darting in and out among the sheltering leaves. The fragrance of lilacs in full bloom is in the air, and I inhale deeply. Brando, our Maine Coon cat, lies curled on the desk besides me, dreaming secret cat dreams, while Sly, the newest addition to our family, dozes on the arm of the love-seat. Mocha lies uncomplainingly in the doorway, patiently awaiting her overdue walk. It is May, 1995, a week shy of my 55th birthday, and my favorite time of year. The harsh, cold, gray winter is finally behind us, and April's month-long showers have helped create the splendor my senses delight in. I feel myself in perfect harmony with this season. Teeming with health and vitality, I am vibrantly alive. As I reflect upon and begin to write about these last three years, my gratitude to God for the gift of my life grows stronger still.

I ask my children, my family, my friends, their memories upon hearing that I am cancer free, for mine are blurred by the emotional intensity I experienced that day.

"What did I say? How did the conversation go?" I inquire. "I can't remember a thing."

They remember. I am laughing and crying. Thanking God. Sounding euphoric. But mostly they remember their own deep sense of relief. The happiness they feel upon hearing the news. Their own laughter and tears. The release of tension from their body. The letting go of fear. Prayers answered. A great miracle manifesting.

Knowing it is an impossible task to call everyone personally without temporarily losing my voice, I write to the hundred plus wonderful people who comprise my healing circle. It is truly a labor of love.

Dear... ,

I am writing you with the joyous news that I AM CANCER FREE. On March 31st, almost a year to the day I was diagnosed with advanced metastasized kidney cancer, I learned that all visible signs of tumor were gone from my body, and that new bone is forming on my ribs. The love, caring, prayers, and healing energies you sent my way played a significant part in bringing this miracle about, and I am deeply grateful to you for your generosity of spirit.

My doctor, who administered the immunotherapy, is literally speechless. He anticipated no change in the tumor for at least two months, based on previous patients' responses to this treatment, and then, only a very gradual and partial regression. I am considered a rarity, that one or two in a hundred to respond this way. He is curious about, and receptive to the alternative forms of healing I employed, so perhaps other patients will benefit from my experience. As for me, I am committed to writing my book *A Year Of Miracles*, about my healing journey from cancer to wholeness. It is my hope that by sharing my story, this book will empower and find its way to those who most need to know that in any given set of circumstances, it is possible to accomplish the seemingly impossible.

After discussion with my doctor, I have agreed to repeat immunotherapy. I view this as an additional life insurance policy as well as a booster vaccine. As I see it, this is a case where more is better than less. I will be in treatment from May 7th through May 14th, at the University of Michigan Medical Center. Once again, I am asking you to focus love, light, and healing energies my way, and once again I thank you.

My life is filled to overflowing. Each day I awaken with joy in my heart, and a smile on my lips. I make preparations for my wedding on July 12th, with gratitude and the expectation of living a long, healthy, happy life with Stan, the man I adore. I am filled with love for God, Stan, my children, family and friends. I am fully and truly alive.

IN LOVE AND LIGHT,
Susan

With the second round of immunotherapy, I learn that Interleukin 2 has a cumulative effect, meaning the adverse side effects are greater each time. No doubt, this is partly due to the fact that the dosage is doubled. The week spent in the hospital is very difficult. I feel lethargic and dull, queasy, frequently nauseous, itchy to the point of distraction, achy, and sore. I retain twenty pounds of fluids, develop ringing in my ears, experience hallucinations and strangely disturbing dreams. It does not help to hear that Dr. Chang recommends a full year of treatment, and if I comply, this is only treatment number two out of a total of four.

"Studies show, Susan, that the select group of patients who have a complete remission and follow the protocol for a year, seldom have a recurrence," Dr. Chang emphatically states.

"That's pretty powerful ammunition," I think, as I hear myself agreeing to a third treatment in September.

A YEAR OF MIRACLES

Stan's father dies of cancer halfway through my second round of immunotherapy. A grieving son flies to Philadelphia to bury his father, while trying to be of comfort to his distraught mother. Unable to be with Stan and support him in his loss, we make do with long nightly phone conversations. Natalie takes it upon herself to visit me during the remainder of my hospital stay, something I fully appreciate, knowing how difficult this generous act is for her to perform. A bond of friendship slowly, tentatively, begins to emerge.

Sharon graduates the School of Social Work, and a month later she and Chuck relocate to the Florida Keys, where new and exciting careers, coupled with the sun, the sea, and the tropical climate lure them. They move with four of their five cats, but concern about the heat becoming too intense for a long- haired cat like Brando, prompts them to leave him with a more than willing me.

Once again, I become aware of how the synergy of Divine Intervention has made a terrifying time that much easier to bear. After living for five years in Los Angeles, Sharon and Chuck have returned to Ann Arbor a mere six months before my bout with cancer begins. They leave barely two months after my complete recovery from cancer. There is no doubt in my mind that Sharon's need to be with her mother during that traumatic year was every bit as strong as my need to have my daughter within arms reach. I am convinced that a loving God with Infinite Wisdom created the circumstances which allowed that miracle to blossom.

The night before my CAT scan, which is scheduled two weeks before our wedding day, I have another significant dream. I see a bright light moving across a clear board. I intuitively know it is a CAT scan, and that it is clear.

Suddenly, a booming voice orders, "write it down," and a pad and pen appear before me.

"There is no evidence of…" the voice says, and uses two words I am unfamiliar with.

To my ears, the words sound like some form of medical terminology.

"I don't understand," I say uncomprehendingly.

The voice, sounding authoritative and somewhat exasperated responds,
"YOU SHOULD KNOW BY NOW. THERE IS NO EVIDENCE OF CANCER ANYWHERE IN YOUR BODY. WRITE IT DOWN."

At that moment, my alarm rings. I drink the hypaque I am required to ingest for the CAT scan, and leave trusting that I am cancer free. Most importantly, when I recall this message around subsequent scans, my anxiety diminishes, and I feel trusting that all will go well. CAT scans can still invoke varying degrees of uneasiness, but as the years pass and I continue to enjoy excellent health, my anxiety level continues to diminish with each scan I have.

July 12, 1992, surrounded by our children, our family, our friends, Stan and I celebrate our love, and join our lives together under God. Marilyn is my maid of honor. Sharon, Elyssa, Natalie and Susan are my bridal attendants. Ari proudly serves as best man for his father. Brent, Kal, Chuck, and Stan's brother Ed are his groomsmen. Tracy is soloist, and sings three songs in her exquisite voice. Pat and June each perform a reading. Our friend Tom plays the flute, accompanied on classical guitar. At last the long awaited moment arrives, and with hearts overflowing with love, joy, and gratitude, Stan and I recite the wedding vows we have written for this special day.

Our Wedding Vows

Susan:
> *Because you share my laughter and my tears, and your belief in me and love help me to heal ...*

Stan:
> *Because you are there to listen and care when I need a friend ...*

Susan:
> *Because your honesty and openness makes it easy for me to trust and love again, and colors my world a safer place ...*

A YEAR OF MIRACLES

Stan:

Because you open my days to sunshine, happiness, warmth, and unbounded joy ...

Susan:

Because your gentle, tender, loving ways, support me in becoming all I can be ...

Stan:

Because your faith and courage inspire me to enjoy my life to its fullest ...

Together:

For all these reasons and more, we choose to join our lives together, on this day, forevermore.

Stan:

I believe the song of world unity begins with the harmony of marriage.

Susan:

I believe we are destined to always be together, and our marriage is part of a far greater plan.

Stan:

I believe the melody of your laughter, and the sparkle of your smile, brings out the child in me.

Susan:

I believe the glee in your eyes, your eagerness to play, and your love of adventure, keeps me forever young.

Stan:

I believe the glow of our love will illuminate all the days and nights of our lives.

Susan:

I believe the sacredness of our love will nourish our souls for all of eternity.

220

Together:

> *We believe the light of God's love blesses our marriage, and our trust in God's love guides us and protects us.*

Susan:

> *I promise to celebrate my love for you, to be joy to your heart and music to your soul.*

Stan:

> *I promise to always value our relationship above all others.*

Susan:

> *I promise to let you know when you please me, to forgive you when you offend me, and to be compassionate in your times of need.*

Stan:

> *I promise to respect your individuality and to support you in becoming all you can be.*

Susan:

> *I promise to keep the magic of our marriage alive, to journey with you wherever the path may lead, knowing love is always our final destination.*

Stan:

> *I promise to hold each day of our marriage precious, to delight in our togetherness and return to you refreshed when we are apart.*

Susan:

> *I promise to nourish you with my willingness, to affirm you with my faith, and to always know God's love in the miracle of you.*

Stan:

> *I promise to always see you in God's beautifying light, to cherish your goodness, and to accommodate our differences in a spirit of love.*

A YEAR OF MIRACLES

Together:

> *These are our heartfelt promises. These are*
> *our sacred vows... to love fully and completely... until*
> *the end of time... forever and a day.*

At our reception we hold a candle lighting ceremony, where we call upon family and friends to join with us, and light one of the eighteen candles.

"In Hebrew," Stan says to our guests, "the number eighteen represents life. Therefore, at this ceremony we will be lighting a circle of eighteen candles as part of our celebration of love and life. Each candle also symbolizes a quality that Susan and I believe keeps the flames of our love burning brightly."

Stan and I alternate calling upon the people we wish to honor, having them light a candle representative of a quality we perceive in them. The eighteen qualities we choose are:

Joy
Forgiveness
Communication
Tenderness
Adventure
Patience
Faith
Trust
Compassion
Gratitude
Flexibility
Courage
Laughter
Spontaneity
Honesty
Willingness
Wisdom
Healing

"The eighteenth candle of healing completes the circle before us," I say, "but since a circle is never ending, it begins again with the candle of joy. It is very meaningful for Stan, myself, and many among us, that this joyous celebration of love and life is taking place today, all because of a miraculous healing. There are two healers in this room, who have contributed in large measure to that healing, and we wish to honor them today. I would like to call upon Dr. Alfred Chang and Dr. James Thomas to join Stan and me in lighting the eighteenth candle of healing."

Sharon stands up, and enthusiastically begins to applaud. As I look around the carriage house, our guests rise as one. Loud applause reverberates throughout the room, as side by side, Dr. Thomas and Dr. Chang light the candle of healing.

When the applause finally ceases, Stan speaks the following words.

"The center candle, encircled by the eighteen candles of life, represents the greatest blessing for Susan and myself. The blessing of our beloved children. Will Sharon, Elyssa, Brent, Natalie and Ari join us in lighting the candle of family."

Stan and I address our five children, and there is both laughter and tears. As the center candle is lit, our lives as a newly formed family begins.

On July 13, 1992, we are married for a second time in a traditional Orthodox Jewish Ceremony performed by Rabbi Goldstein. This is a smaller wedding, attended only by our closest family, friends, and members of the Chabad House congregation. The ceremony takes place outdoors under a Chuppah, a canopy which is held over a Jewish bride and groom by their four honor attendants. I am unfamiliar with, and lack an understanding of many of the rituals and prayers that are part of the ceremony, but I fully understand how important it is to Stan that we be married in this religious ceremony. And for that reason, it also becomes important to me. The contrast between the two weddings is unmistakable, but the basic similarities of joy, love, and heartfelt blessings are abundantly present at both. Especially powerful is the sense of being held in God's embrace as we recite our vows.

Talking with Esther Goldstein at our reception, and observing her happiness, I recall the day she visited at the hospital, shortly after my kidney surgery. This modest, intelligent woman, who derives great pleasure in doing mitzvahs [good deeds] for others, organized the women of the sisterhood, and with her children in tow, walked five miles each way on the Sabbath to see me. Climbing the seven flights of steps to my hospital room to pray for my healing, and delivering words of encouragement born from her deep abiding faith that Hashem [God] would be merciful towards me, the presence of Esther and the others raised my spirits. Now, prayers answered, a smiling Esther sings and dances as she celebrates our marriage.

A week later, Stan and I leave in Morph for a seven week honeymoon that will take us to Glacier National Park, Banff, Jasper, Vancouver, Vancouver Island, and on a two day boat trip through the inner passage to Prince Rupert, 30 miles outside of Alaska.

On August 10th, three months to the day after Stan's father's death, his mother Syd joins her beloved husband. We fly in a daze from Vancouver to Philadelphia for the funeral, and remain a week while Stan and his brother Ed sit Shiva. [a prescribed period of mourning] Both sons takes comfort in the thought their parents are reunited, something which their mother had yearned for since the day her husband died. We return to Vancouver and continue our honeymoon in a subdued state of mind. Arriving home in mid-September, I enter the hospital shortly thereafter, for my third round of immunotherapy.

I have forgotten the side effects of immunotherapy are at their worst once all treatment has ceased. Upon being discharged from the hospital and returning home, I remember all too well.

"I don't want to undergo a fourth and final round of immunotherapy in January," I tell Stan unhappily. "I need to believe three treatments will be as effective as four. Unless I do, I know that I will subject myself to this one last time."

"Let's meet with Dr. Chang in December, and decide then," Stan suggests soothingly.

Dr. Chang is candid with us. "There is no set schedule, but we do try to treat up to a year," he explains. "Nor is there a real rationale as to how much to treat, especially for complete responses."

"Can you give me a compelling reason to continue treatment, and put myself through all the discomfort again?" I bluntly ask.

"Other than my own personal opinion that more is better than less, I can't. If you decide in favor of a fourth round of immunotherapy, I would treat you with a lower dosage. However, the final choice is yours. Think about it, and get back with me after the New Year."

I know my answer before we leave.

"I am done," I say to Stan on the short drive home. "No more treatments. I have trust in my healing and faith it will continue. This part of my journey is complete. I envision moving into the New Year steeped in the teachings that have come as a result of my healing journey, filled with a fullness, love, and purpose that will continue to guide me."

Stan squeezes my hand, and smiles at me.

"I totally support your decision," he lovingly says.

Over dinner we share future visions of our life's work. We speak enthusiastically about those projects we will collaborate on, and those we will accomplish individually. The future stretches before us unencumbered. God is watching over us, and we know ourselves to be blessed.

1993 is a year of new beginnings. I begin this book, surprised at the many starts and stops along the way. Anything I have managed to avoid during my year long healing journey from cancer, I am now afforded the opportunity to grapple with. It is not a matter of choice. It is an absolute necessity as repressed fears, sadness, pain and grief rise to the surface, are dealt with, and released. I come to understand that the act of writing this book brings with it the gift of a complete healing. I am tender and gentle with myself, a loving mother to my wounded child, as my full range of emotions tumbles forth. I write when I can. I cry when I must. I process when I need to. I embrace life fully and with renewed vigor. I turn to Stan for nurturance. He unfailingly nourishes and encourages me. I live in the moment, and persevere.

We celebrate Jennifer and Jon's wedding in February, and I proudly stand besides her on that special day, as her "other mother." I have fulfilled the promise to Jennifer's mother Marilyn, which I made shortly before her death. I can feel her joyful presence as it permeates her daughter's wedding day. Twenty months later beautiful Marilyn Jo is born, and with her birth I become a first time, doting grandmother.

In August, Elyssa and Jeff purchase her childhood home from me, and in September she begins a four year evening MBA program at the University of Michigan School of Business. Amidst turbulent emotions, I dismantle my home of seventeen years, and Stan and I move into our new home, his previous residence. After extensive renovations, we transform it into a bright, open, airy, welcoming home radiating peace and tranquillity. This home I now reside in, has become a composite of both of us, and I find myself growing to love it. It is in my study, surrounded by my crystals, paintings, angel collection, photographs, and plants, that I sit at the desk I share with Brando, and during the next eighteen months bring this book to completion.

In December 1993 Brent and Tracy graduate from the University of Michigan. Tracy leaves for the bright lights of New York City, seeking fame and fortune in musical theater. At her first audition, she is offered a one year contract to play Gumby and Lady Griddlebone in the European tour of CATS. An ecstatic Tracy returns home in March to pack for Europe, and visit with family and friends. After a large farewell party, Tracy leaves Ann Arbor for rehearsals in Switzerland. In April 1995, after a spectacular one year tour with CATS, Tracy auditions for Les Miserables. She is promptly hired, and signs a fifteen month contract which begins November, 1995. The show will open in January 1996 in Duisburg, Germany, and will remain there for its entire run. After touring Switzerland, Germany, Austria, and Italy, Tracy is thrilled to have a place to call home for a year, and looks forward to renting an apartment, and acquiring a cat. Just as Stan and I flew to Milan, Italy to see Tracy perform in CATS, we are planning a trip to Duisburg, Germany to see Tracy in Les Miserables.

While applying to law schools for Fall 1994 admission, Brent is required to write a personal statement, detailing an experience that has had a profound impact on his life. What he writes moves me to tears, and I ask for and receive his permission to include it in this book. I find Brent's writing to be inspiring, filled with wisdom, and some very basic truths.

Brent's Personal Statement

During my sophomore year at the University of Michigan, my mother was diagnosed with cancer. She was told that it had spread throughout her body, and that she would have less than a 5 percent chance of surviving. She was told to get her affairs in order. When I was told of this news, the thing that stood out for me the most, was the less than 5 percent chance she was given to survive. Initially, what this meant to me, were that my days with her were limited, and that I would need to savor the remaining time we had left together.

Yet when my mother received this news, she did not take the pessimistic view that I now look back upon myself as taking. She spoke to me, my sisters, and her friends in a reassuring tone. She told us that she needed all of our support, and that with it she would triumph in the face of adversity. She said that by having a strong faith in God and herself, by using a prayer circle consisting of family and friends, by employing conventional and alternative healing techniques, as well as a great deal of positive energy, it would only be a matter of time until she overcame this challenge in her life. Because of the great faith she asked each of us to instill in her and ourselves, I found my own belief system being challenged.

Throughout the next several months, I found myself questioning the initial beliefs that I had concerning my mother's illness. Through being inspired by her and those around her, along with the great deal of progress she began to make, my understanding of how to cope with adversity was slowly redefined. I saw how she took control of a situation, which I had assumed was one in which little could be done. In the end, when her final visit to the doctor's office confirmed no traces of cancer, I discovered a newly created belief system within myself.

From my mother's effort to overcome cancer, I learned a lesson about myself. I found that in order to look beyond the facts of trying circumstances, it not only takes faith in yourself, but the need for others to have faith in you as well. When I saw how her strength and the efforts of the healing circle contributed to her well being, I began to understand the importance of using my own strength to overcome adversity in my life. I developed an awareness that when faced with trying circumstances in the future, I would use the trust within myself, as well as the support of my friends and family, to work through these circumstances.

I feel that I can honestly say that this episode with my mother, and the effect it had on me, is one that will change my life forever. Two years after my mother's bout with cancer, these new found qualities proved successful, when I was forced to call upon them for myself. During this time, I experienced a very difficult episode in my own life. However, I found that I was able to develop a way of experiencing and then overcoming this episode, by using my own inner strength and the support of those around me.

Brent has been accepted at four law schools, and has chosen to attend the University of Denver, where he has just completed his first year. During his limited free time, he rock climbs, mountain bikes, camps, hikes, and skis. He is seriously considering a joint law/social work degree, specializing in public interest law, and working on behalf of neglected and abused children. It is clear to me, that wherever Brent focuses his considerable talents, there will be many who will benefit from his humanitarian approach, inner strength, ongoing efforts, and strongly ingrained belief system.

In August 1994, Sharon and Chuck fulfill a dream of theirs, and buy a sprawling ranch home in a quiet residential neighborhood in Key West. It is a bicycle ride away from Sharon's job as a child therapist with emotionally disturbed children, and is equally close to the Navy base where Chuck is employed as a marriage and family counselor. Stan and I visit twice in less than a year, and we dream of a time in the not too distant future, when we will reside in Key West during the long, cold, gray, Michigan winters.

Natalie, is a very talented film maker with a nationally and internationally acclaimed award winning documentary, "One Banana, Two Bananas," which chronicles her mother Lynne's courageous battle with MS. She has recently made her debut as director of a full length feature film. Natalie lives in Chicago, and will be completing her studies in Film and Video at Columbia College next spring. With the aid of a generous grant, she is hard at work on her most recent documentary, a study of women and their relationship to their breasts. As for our relationship, it has undergone a complete metamorphosis, a one hundred and eighty degree turn. Natalie and I are as close and loving now as we once were distant and separate, and the change is one that sustains, nourishes and benefits us both. I am delighted that Natalie, in her own words is happy to be, "one of my kids."

Ari, a senior at Western Michigan University, is majoring in biomedical sciences. Inspired by my healing, and strongly influenced by the death of his beloved mother from MS, a still incurable disease, he plans to obtain a graduate degree and make his contribution as a researcher in the field of biomedical sciences. Ari's long range dream is to discover a cure for a presently incurable disease. If it happens to be MS or Cancer so much the better, but he is not limiting his sights. Upon graduating Ari plans to relocate to Colorado, to be near his best friend and stepbrother Brent, and begin pursuing his lofty goals. Stan and I look forward to visiting our sons, to ski with them in winter, to hike and camp with them in summer, but most importantly of all, to share quality family time together.

A joyous celebration awaits us, as preparations for the July 15th wedding that will unite Elyssa and Jeff seven short weeks from now, nears completion. Sharon and Chuck, Brent, Ari, Natalie, and Tracy will soon be under our roof, filling our home again with love, laughter, and the exuberant vibrancy of youth. For much too short a time, our family will be reunited before scattering in five completely different directions again. These are the comings and goings of our family, and though each coming together is followed by a going away, at the end of each going away, is another coming together. In knowing this, good-byes are made easier, for there always is that next hello to look forward to.

If I had but one wish for Elyssa and Jeff on their wedding day, it would be that their marriage be similar to ours, in the sense that they grow ever closer and more deeply in love with each passing day. Stan and I will be celebrating our third wedding anniversary, and I awaken every morning grateful to be married to him, thankful he is lying besides me, and eager to share with him whatever the new day holds. We are living our wedding vows just as we envisioned, and our life together is all we ever dreamed it could be, and more.

This golden life I am privileged to be living is what I fought so determinedly for during a full year that began with a diagnosis of a fatal disease, and ended with a complete and miraculous healing. The vision of what could be, kept my spirit alive and ever hopeful, energizing me, and creating an innate ability to bounce back quickly. After two initial periods of devastation, the first brought about upon learning I had cancer, and the second upon learning six months later that the cancer had recurred, I was able to do just that. I am convinced this ability to bounce back was crucial to my complete recovery.

Though in many ways, my soul's journey was one in which I had no choice but to journey alone, I seldom felt alone. Being blessed with Stan, my children, my family, my friends, and my physicians' love, support, encouragement, and intrinsic belief in me, affirmed and strengthened my resolve to do all in my power to heal into life. Without this support, my journey may have had a very different outcome. If you are reading this book and have cancer or any other life threatening illness, please don't underestimate the importance of a loving support system, and do all in your power to create one. It can make a significant difference in your ability to heal.

Having cancer, even in my worst moments, when I raged and pleaded with God, felt sorry for myself, and grieved my likely demise, brought also the gift of a unique opportunity to look death squarely in the eye, face my mortality head on, and grow from the encounter. I began to understand on a soul level the words of the woman who said, "cancer is a gift for the woman who has everything." Faced with probable death, I reached deep inside myself, past illusions of who I was, past beliefs of my own true nature, past definitions both of society's making, and my own. When I merged with my essential essence, only then did I discover the wholeness that has always been within, and recognize myself for who I really am, a cherished child of God. In living my essence, and my wholeness, through daily words and deeds, I do honor to myself and others, find meaning in all I do, experience unrelenting gratitude, because there is always something to be grateful for, and feel ever more closely aligned with God.

Life is brighter, richer, more vibrant, more joyous, and my appreciation is fuller, deeper, and more intense. I love more, and express it freely and frequently. I savor each day with a childlike simplicity, as an adventure to be lived with wonder and awe. I stop often, not only to smell the roses, but to plant rose bushes of my own making, so that during my lifetime, and long after I am gone, the fragrance will linger on the air, bringing pleasure to others. I don't put off for tomorrow, for I know there is only today, only the present moment to engage in fully. I laugh, and then laugh some more, for it is true that laughter heals, and you can't overdose on it, no matter how frequently you use it. Would I have arrived here without the gifts of cancer? I would like to think so, but I honestly can't say. For me at least, facing my death brought with it the heightened appreciation of life with all its nuances, its joys and sorrows, the whole cacophony of the human experience.

I take better care of my body by feeding it healthy foods, and exercising it regularly, and it repays me by looking and feeling good, and remaining in perfect health. I look upon my body as the vehicle that houses my soul, and treat it with the same respect, love, and care, I would lavish on any house I live in. It serves me well, and deserves only the best. I usually lead with my heart, knowing it to be the home of my spirit, as well as the bridge between my body and mind, and experience increased clarity, cooperation and harmony whenever I do. The gift from cancer, the pearl in the oyster, once gained cannot be lost. Misplaced occasionally, but quickly retrieved. Cherished even more for its temporary absence.

The gift extends into all of my relationships, from my nearest and dearest, to the overwhelmed, angry client who enters my office seeking relief. I behold each person as part of my family, another child of God, and speak kind, encouraging words when I can, while opening myself as a source of love flowing their way. I have been shown how healing and transformative the power of love can be, and the miracles that occur in the lives of those who open to it. Surely, my own healing was made possible through the love sent by others, and received by me. Like so many other women, it was easier for me to nurture others, rather than receiving needed nurturance myself. However, these days I find I am more evenly balanced in giving and receiving, as the yin and the yang integrate.

My spirituality, and my relationship with God have undergone the most significant change of all. It was easy to talk the spiritual talk, and affirm my belief in the goodness of God, when despite the ups and downs of my life, I was free of life threatening trauma. But with the occurrence of cancer, unexposed doubts and fears surfaced, and my faith and trust were continually challenged. What was my relationship to God? And God's to me? Could I still believe in God's love for me? God's desire for my highest good? Could I still hold firm in my faith, even with a recurrence? Could I surrender into Divine Purpose, and make peace with it? What if instead of healing into life as I so desperately desired, I would heal into death as some do? Could I will to will God's Will? Could I trust in God as the source of all good, whatever the outcome? As I grappled with these questions and others, I was delighted to find my faith muscle growing stronger, and my ongoing relationship with God blossoming, and becoming the pivotal point around which the rest of my life evolves. By moving out of my own way, through a heartfelt acceptance of, and surrender to, a Will so much greater than my own, a much more meaningful healing than I had ever envisioned became my reality. The healing of my body, mind, and spirit. My healing into wholeness, through the discovery of my True Self.

I close this book in the hope that it touches you in ways that will inspire and empower you on your journey toward healing and wholeness. May the miracle of my healing continue to reach out as a reminder, at those times you most need to remember, that it is possible to accomplish the seemingly impossible.

A YEAR OF MIRACLES

RECOMMENDED READING

Achterberg, Jeanne: *Imagery in Healing.* Boston: Shambhala, 1985.

Achterberg, Jeanne; Dossey, Barbara and Kolkmeier, Leslie: *Rituals of Healing.* New York: Bantam, 1994.

Anderson, Greg: *The Cancer Conqueror.* Kansas City: Andrews and McMeel, 1988.

Bloch, Richard and Annette: *Cancer...there's hope.* Kansas City: R.A. Bloch Cancer Foundation, 1982. [Available without cost. Call 1-800-4-CANCER.]

Bloch, Annette and Richard: *Fighting Cancer.* R.A. Bloch Cancer Foundation, 1985. [Available without cost. Call 1-800-4-CANCER or 816-932-8453.]

Block, Shira: *Step-By-Step Miracles.* New York: Kensington, 1995.

Borysenko, Joan: *Minding the Body, Mending the Mind.* New York: Bantam, 1988.

Chaitow, Leon: *The Body/Mind Purification Program.* New York: Simon and Schuster, 1990.

Chopra, Deepak: *Quantum Healing: Exploring the Frontiers of Mind/Body Medicine.* New York: Bantam Books, 1989.

Cousins, Norman: *Anatomy of an Illness.* New York: Norton and Company, Inc. 1979.

Cousins, Norman: *Head First: The Biology of Hope.* New York: E.P. Dutton, 1989.

Davis, Bruce and Wright Davis, Genny: *The Heart of Healing.* New York. Bantam, 1985.

Dossey, Larry: *Healing Words.* New York: Harper Collins, 1993.

East West Foundation, Fawcett, Ann and Smith, Cynthia: *Cancer Free.* Tokyo and New York: Japan Publications, Inc. 1991

Engstrand, Beatrice C: *The Gift of Healing.* New York: Wynwood Press, 1990.

Fritz, Robert: *The Path of Least Resistance.* New York: Ballantine, 1989.

Hay, Louise L: *You Can Heal Your Life.* California: Hay House, 1984.

Hirshberg, Caryle and O'Regan, Brendan: *Spontaneous Remission: An Annotated Bibliography.* Sausalito: Institute of Noetic Sciences, 1993.

Hirshberg, Caryle and Barasch, Marc Ian: *Remarkable Recovery.* New York: Riverhead Books, 1995.

Kushner, Harold S: *When Bad Things Happen To Good People.* New York: Schocken Books, 1981.

Lawlis, G. Frank: *The Cure.* California: Resource Publications, Inc. 1994.

Lazaris: *The Sacred Journey: You and Your Higher Self.* California: Concept: Synergy Publishing. 1987.

LeShan, Lawrence: *How to Meditate.* New York: Bantam, 1975.

LeShan, Lawrence: *You Can Fight for Your Life: Emotional Factors in the Treatment of Cancer.* New York: M. Evans, 1977.

LeShan, Lawrence: *Cancer as a Turning Point.* New York: Dutton, 1989.

Levine, Stephen: *Healing Into Life And Death.* New York: Doubleday, 1987.

RECOMMENDED READING

Levine, Stephen: *Guided Meditations, Explorations and Healings.* New York: Doubleday, 1991.

Moen, Larry: *Meditations for Healing.* Florida: United States Publishing, 1994.

Moss, Ralph: *Cancer Therapy, The Independent Consumer's Guide to Nontoxic Treatment and Prevention.* New York: Equinox Press, 1995.

Nessim, Susan and Ellis, Judith: *Cancervive.* New York: Houghton Mifflin, 1991.

Rosenberg, Steven A. and Barry, John M.: *The Transformed Cell.* New York: G.P. Putnam's Sons, 1992.

Shattock, E.H.: *A Manual of Self-Healing.* Vermont: Destiny Books, 1982.

Siegel, Bernie S.: *Love, Medicine and Miracles.* New York: Harper and Row, 1986.

Siegel, Bernie S.: *Peace, Love and Healing.* New York: Harper and Row, 1989.

Siegel, Bernie S.: *How To Live Between Office Visits.* New York: Harper Collins, 1993.

Simonton, O. Carl, Matthews-Simonton, Stephanie and Creighton, James L.: *Getting Well Again.* New York: Bantam, 1978.

Simonton, O. Carl, Henson, Reid and Hampton Brenda: *The Healing Journey.* New York: Bantam, 1992.

Smith, Harry Douglas: *The Secret of Instantaneous Healing.* New York: Parker Publishing Company, 1965.

Tate, David A.: *Health, Hope, And Healing.* New York: M. Evans & Company, 1989.

Wadler, Joyce: *My Breast.* New York: Addison-Wesley, 1992.

Walters, Richard: *Options, The Alternative Cancer Therapy Book.* New York: Avery Publishing Group Inc., 1993.

Weil, Andrew: *Health And Healing.* Boston: Houghton Mifflin, 1985.

Weil, Andrew: *Spontaneous Healing.* New York: Alfred A. Knopf, 1995.

Wilde, Stuart: *Miracles.* New Mexico: White Dove International, Inc., 1988.

Williams, Wendy: *The Power Within.* New York: Simon & Schuster, 1991.

ADDITIONAL RESOURCES

Fight for Your Life, is a two and a half hour video, that teaches those with cancer how to become involved in their healing process. It offers hope to patients and their families in the fight for life, and can be ordered by calling, 1-800-888-5236.

Silent Unity believes in the power of affirmative prayer. They are available around the clock to pray with you, and to keep faith with you. There is never a charge, and each call is treated with reverence and confidentiality. Write *Silent Unity*, 1901 NW Blue Parkway, Unity Village, MO 64065-0001. Or call: (816) 246-5400. If you have an urgent need and have no means of paying for the call, you may call *Silent Unity* toll free at 1-800-669-7729. The toll free number is only for calls originating in the United States.

The Lighthouse Center, Inc., founded by Catherine "Chetana" Florida, is a non-profit charitable organization dedicated to spiritual development through mantra meditation, chanting, and prayer. In addition, various classes and workshops to accelerate spiritual growth are offered throughout the year. Write: *The Lighthouse Center*, Inc. P.O. Box 645, Whitmore Lake, MI 48189. Or call: (313) 449-0611.

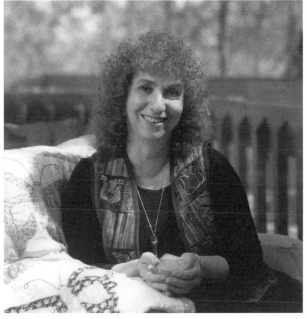

Photo by D. C. Goings

Susan Wolf Sternberg, co-founder of Tapestry Counseling and Consulting Center, is a psychotherapist in private practice since 1976. Working in a gentle, supportive, non judgmental manner she assists clients in creating beneficial changes in their lives. Since healing from cancer, Susan has specialized in working with individuals with life threatening illness. Helping them discover their unique strengths and abilities, she encourages them to apply the full force of that power to their own healing journey. She also facilitates Healing from Cancer Empowerment Groups and Weekend Workshops. A natural born storyteller who is popular with audiences, she is an inspirational speaker.

Susan loves the great outdoors. Hiking the mountains, walking the forest paths, meditating at the seashore, she feels most deeply connected with her spirituality. The mother of three grown children, Susan lives in Ann Arbor, Michigan with her husband and soulmate Stan, their two cats Brando and Sly, and yellow Labrador Retriever puppy Gaia. Having written since childhood, she is now at work on a book of vignettes, that encompasses the experiences, teachings, lessons, and wisdom she has gleaned during her first fifty five years of life.

Susan can be reached through Star Mountain Press, PO Box 1845, Ann Arbor, MI, 48106.

TO ORDER

A Year of Miracles

If you would like additional copies of *A Year of Miracles* to share with family and friends, they can be ordered directly from Star Mountain Press. The cost is $13.95 per book plus $4.00 postage and handling for up to two books. Add $1.00 additional postage and handling for each book over two books. Please send check or money order to:

Star Mountain Press
Post Office Box 1845
Ann Arbor, MI 48106

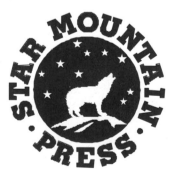